TRY TO REMEMBER

TRY TO REMEMBER

Judith Freeland

iUniverse, Inc.

New York Lincoln Shanghai

TRY TO REMEMBER

iUniverse books may be ordered through booksellers or by contacting:

iUniverse
2021 Pine Lake Road, Suite 100
Lincoln, NE 68512
www.iuniverse.com
1-800-Authors (1-800-288-4677)

ISBN-13: 978-0-595-37844-9 (pbk)
ISBN-13: 978-0-595-82218-8 (ebk)
ISBN-10: 0-595-37844-7 (pbk)
ISBN-10: 0-595-82218-5 (ebk)

Printed in the United States of America

In loving memory of Raymond Orlando Gregerson (June 1, 1905–June 4, 1992), this book is dedicated to those who share his heritage.

Contents

September, 1986–September 1987 Before the Nursing Home

CHAPTER 1   "Senile Old Fool"?. 3

September 1987–September 1988 Nursing Home: First Year

CHAPTER 2   Chatting 15

September 1988–September 1989 Nursing Home: Second Year

CHAPTER 3   Come to Visit 27

CHAPTER 4   College, Courtship, and Children 34

CHAPTER 5   Perky Voices 44

September 1989–September 1990 Nursing Home: Third Year

CHAPTER 6   Share This With Me 57

CHAPTER 7   Memory is Not Linear. 64

CHAPTER 8   Horses and Holidays 71

September 1990–September 1991 Nursing Home: Fourth Year

CHAPTER 9   Windows. 83

CHAPTER 10   A Home of Their Own 92

CHAPTER 11   Who? Where? When? 100

CHAPTER 12   Time Like a River 106

September 1991–June 1992 Nursing Home: Fifth Year

CHAPTER 13   Nightmares and Fairy Tales 113

CHAPTER 14   He Used to Know Them 119

CHAPTER 15   Home. 126

AFTERWORD 127

September, 1986– September 1987 Before the Nursing Home

"Don't forget to remember not to forget."
—Johnny Hart

1

"SENILE OLD FOOL"?

The words hurt. He probably was not meant to hear his neighbor muttering "Senile old fool, barely remembers his own name, most likely." Greg thought he had seen the man before, but he wasn't sure, so he had politely introduced himself before commenting on what a lovely day it was and continuing his morning walk.

Greg preferred solitary walks, meeting no one whose name or face he might be supposed to know. He cherished striding across the acres of pasture land surrounding his home, skirting the low spiky green bushes that he thought were chaparral; circling the huge Torrey pines, their sinuous trunks creeping along the ground before rearing up in shapes like dinosaurs, their funny little, bright red blossoms looking more like pine cones than flowers; and stepping over or around the sagebrush, Queen Anne's Lace (yarrow, really) and yellow or white daisies rioting randomly on land only he and the occasional cow ever frequented.

Usually, he went beyond the pastures into the scrubby woods, very different from the moisture-rich woods of Minnesota and Manitoba. If he had stuck to the woods, and not crossed the road, thinking to explore new pastures and woodlands, he would not have been embarrassed by the abrupt appearance of those two men he would later realize had been his neighbors.

There was nothing wrong with his memory. There was just so very much to remember after 81 years of living. He had perfectly clear memories. Looking at his watch, he remembered that he was supposed to drive into town for the mail. As he walked up to the house, he admired, as he always did, the huge boulders lining the driveway, overhung with the spreading branches of the lone manzanita, now rare even in its native terrain.

He admired the house, too, but frowned momentarily, wondering for the umpteenth time if he and Floy had made a mistake when they had opted for orienting the layout so the living room windows overlooked meadows and woods. The view, never quite the same, was always restful. But guests had to enter the house by the back entry, just off the kitchen, facing a bathroom door that he didn't always remember to shut.

Floy was waiting for him. "After you get the mail, would you stop to pick up a couple limes? Lois and Dick are coming for happy hour, and Mary and Walter. He drinks gin and tonic, but must have it with a slice of lime." He would, Greg thought. Everyone else in their social group drank beer or bourbon or maybe scotch. A man whose tweed jacket sported leather elbow patches would have to be different. With gin and tonic in hand—with its slice of lime—Walter had never, until recently, let a discussion go by without reminding everyone that he was working on the eighth edition of his best-selling history text book for high schoolers.

Since Floy had ever so casually let it slip that her daughter the college professor had published a college text book and two other, more scholarly books, the eighth edition of whatever it was called had not been mentioned. Everyone really liked Mary, and apart from his occasional pomposity, Walter was an interesting, well-informed person, so the two were frequent guests.

Greg said he would remember to get limes. He didn't tell her about his embarrassing encounter with the neighbors, or that he'd forgotten about the mail.

As he left the post office, he had a feeling there was something else he was supposed to do. Couldn't have been very important, and he was ready to go home. But this road didn't look familiar. How could he have gone the wrong way in the tiny town of Julian, California? It wasn't much more than a post office, where people like him who lived in the surrounding hills collected their mail and bought a few groceries. There was a school, just around the corner. Maybe if he parked here while the children got safely across the road, he could remember the way home.

The car radio was on, and Harry Bellafonte was singing "Try to remember…" Greg muttered "Never mind a time in September; I'm trying to remember how to get home!"

Evidently the last bell had rung: kids were boiling out the school doors, boisterous packs of boys running, whirling, jumping as if the Pamplona bulls were on their heels, and small groups, often just pairs, of girls, whispering and giggling to each other as they drifted toward the waiting parade of Cadillacs, Lincolns, the odd Ford, a very snazzy red convertible—foreign car—and three pickup trucks. The few town kids waited at the corner for the crossing guard to snap up her STOP sign and march to the middle of the road to halt any traffic that might appear.

There were no crossing guards when he was a boy, no lineup of cars driven by doting parents, no traffic to avoid, just the occasional horse with rider or buggy attached. He and his classmates had walked the couple blocks or couple miles to their homes. He had loved school, where he had acquired his lifelong love of reading. He remembered fulfilling his wish of reading every book in the town library. There weren't that many of them.

He hadn't read a book in a while. Had he forgotten how to read? No, he could read the sign in front of the car, "Yield to pedestrians in crosswalk." Oh, sure, this was the grade school, and to get home he just had to turn left at the next corner and stay on that road until his turn. Why had he forgotten that? He had overheard Dr. Mazur saying something about Alzheimer's during his checkup last month. Ray MacKenzie caught Alzheimer's when he was only 54, and had to quit his accounting job because he couldn't remember numbers. Greg counted to 25. No problem. And he was retired, anyway.

But forgetting his way home, even for a minute, bothered him. He had lost his way before, but never in everyday surroundings.

Last year, Larry had invited him to his home in Phoenix for a few days of golf. Greg hadn't played any golf in the last couple summers at the lake, and he was looking forward to some time with his son, doing what they both enjoyed.

The drive from Julian to Phoenix should have been an easy eight hour drive, mostly on freeways. He had done the trip to San Diego often enough that the car could probably do it without him. Somehow, he got turned around and was going the wrong way on Interstate 5 and didn't know how to turn back. Finally he took an exit ramp to a service station to ask, and had them write out the directions to get him back on track.

Then he missed the switch from Interstate 5 to Interstate 10, and began to panic. He was low on gas by this time. Another service station, more directions to try to read as he drove. Greg finally found Phoenix, but there were highways and roads and cars going in every direction and he didn't know which direction to take. He pulled to the side of the road and sat, shoulders heaving, struggling not to break down and just bawl. Men don't cry.

The patrol officer was very kind, once he realized Greg was a lost tourist. He looked at Greg's driver's license and his set of directions to Larry's place, told Greg that his son had asked the police to watch for him, and then said, "Just follow me," leading the way to safety. Greg was surprised to learn that the easy eight-hour drive had taken more than twelve. It was after sunset.

Greg shook his head. Anyone could get turned around on unfamiliar roads. Anyone could get confused about how to get where he was going if he hadn't been there before. But he had also had trouble recently getting home from San Diego, a drive he had done many times.

He'd taken Judie to meet friends near the San Diego airport. Maybe he got confused because they hadn't gone to the airport, as was usual after one of her visits. Before his daughter hugged him goodbye, she pointed to the sign "To Interstate 5" about half a block away. So he shouldn't have missed it. Floy was frantic when he got home, and it didn't help matters that he did not know where he had been for five hours.

Maybe his memory really was slipping. He had always known where he was going and how to get there, in uninhabited desert country or busy metropolis. But each time he got confused, he was alone. He had never been lost when Floy was with him.

He remembered driving her to the San Diego hospital. They wouldn't let him stay with her while they removed the infected eye. They told him to go home. He had started to do that, but had turned around and come back to see that she was all right, see if she needed anything. He drove around San Diego for hours, fruitlessly trying to remember how to get to the hospital. Finally, all he could do was to try to find his way home to Julian. He needed a drink.

His beautiful Floy, somewhat vain about her looks—with good reason—with an ugly, raw hole under the bandage. She refused to look in a mirror until the scar healed and the glass eye could be put in. Even after the glass eye restored her looks to normal, she stopped wearing makeup, even lipstick. And she didn't laugh much anymore. Sometimes, he no longer recognized her.

Maybe it was because he was retired now and was home all the time that Floy had said he should go by himself to visit each of the kids. A neighbor had driven him to the airport. Floy could no longer drive, and she had con-

vinced Greg that he should not drive to Phoenix this time; planes were quicker.

He remembered spending a few days in May with Larry in Phoenix. Barb had gone someplace either to give him time alone with his son or—she did like him, didn't she? After the first evening when Larry had too much to drink and he guessed he did, too, he just wanted to go home.

Larry had tried to entertain him. He had taken him to an orange grove and a wild life enclosure and a cascading series of four man-made lakes high up in the mountains, with no trees—just canyons full of cactus. He just wanted to go home, and he was angry at Larry, who said he couldn't do that: he was going to see Judie in Michigan next.

That visit was okay. Judie and Al—he had to keep reminding himself that he had never met Al before. He kept thinking he had. Al looked so familiar. Wasn't he a grown up Otis, a kid he'd gone to school with? Anyway, he liked the guy, and not just because he had horses. Al and Judie—Greg had called her Floy a couple times; so like her mother—they had seemed pleased that he liked to spend a lot of time walking along the horse pasture fences, talking to the horses. But he had really been eager to get home.

Getting off the next plane, he still wasn't home. Larry's younger boy was there, saying they were going to the lake. Well, that would be all right—Floy and Jeannie would be there. Wouldn't they?

Dan, his grandson, wasn't much of a cook, and his concept of a dinner menu was not Greg's. Where was Floy? His wife was supposed to be here. Her meals were properly balanced and properly served. Pizza in a box and parked on the kitchen table with paper plates and paper towels in lieu of napkins would have outraged her. It outraged him.

Greg finally had suggested going to Mooswa for dinner, and asked Dan to phone for reservations. Greg was not eavesdropping. He was in the bathroom. But the phone was just around the corner in the hallway to the kitchen, so he had heard Dan's side of the conversation all too clearly. "Miss Wood, Grandpa wants to come there for dinner...No, it won't be all right. He thinks he still owns the place, and he'll be expecting to be treated like visiting royalty...You're sure? Well, okay, but don't say I didn't warn you."

Greg remembered other dinners at the Mooswa dining room, the dinners of past summers, with Floy graciously responding to the greetings of Les and Edie, the manag-

ers he had hired, and all the staff, who didn't really treat them like visiting royalty, but with the friendly deference due to visiting owners.

Shaking off the day dreams, he ruefully recalled the lengthy negotiations when he had sold Mooswa. Now he was just another visitor on holiday. His holiday in hell, it was becoming.

Finally it was August and he was heading for home, after a seemingly interminable summer, one that had lasted less than a month, at the lake he'd always loved. A summer of wrongness, of gentle memories in conflict with a mean reality. Danny insisted on driving back from the lake to Fargo. Greg had been driving 75,000–100,000 miles a year for over 30 years, and knew he was a safer driver than his grandson, but he was tired of arguing. He was just plain tired.

Pretending to sleep so he wouldn't have to talk to his grandson, he watched the harvest-ready fields pass by his window. He remembered another summer when the hay and wheat fields looked like this, ripening in the sun.

1915

Just after his tenth birthday, as soon as school was out, Greg did what many boys his age from small rural towns did: he hired on with a harvest crew heading for Kansas. They followed the summer northward, working long hours in the fields of Kansas, then Nebraska, South Dakota, and finally North Dakota. They cut the hay at one farm, moved down the road to another farm and then another, then back to the first ones, to build weather-repellent haystacks.

The finished stacks, big as houses, looked like Indian burial mounds, and the kids in the crew enlivened their rare free hours pretending that the ghosts of long-dead Indians were on the warpath again, hot on their heels. Or, risking the wrath of the farmer who hadn't hired a crew to strew his hay all over the ground after stacking it, the youngsters scaled the heights and, pretending to be on skis or fast toboggans, slid screaming down the sides.

A rare few progressive farms had the new baling machines, but every man and child on the crews hated them: the bales had to be hand-tied, and the twine scored the palms of their hands with bloody gashes.

Greg was aware that eventually, someone had invented a machine that both baled and tied, and he liked the tidiness of the precise rows of modern hay bales waiting to be picked up and stored in barns, but he missed the haystacks of his childhood.

Greg loved the sight and sound of the wind blowing through a hay or wheat field, looking and sounding like waves on a distant, golden sea. In a way, it was sad to watch the proud plumes of gold and green fall before the cutting blades, but there was a satisfying orderliness to the separation of grain and chaff, a massive rightness about a haystack. Some farmers had fields of flax, blue as the ocean that he vowed he would see some day. Profitable as this work was, and good for his mind and body, he was not going to spend his life doing empty-minded physical labor on the farms of strangers.

Every day of that first summer, and every day of every summer for the next eight years was the same as the ones before and those that would follow: up before sunrise, then breakfast at the long cookhouse tables loaded with scrambled or fried eggs, crisp bacon, sausages, toast and jam, and coffee. He liked a lot of milk in his coffee. He knew that milk built strong bones and teeth.

Then out to the fields for the work he knew was building the muscles that would make him a man. After four hours of hot, sweaty, chaff-sticky work, they got a short break for water, more coffee, and maybe—at the nicer farms—cookies. They toiled for three more hours, until noon, and then it was time for dinner back at the cookhouse.

The farmers' wives, daughters, neighbors, and other female kin spent their mornings cooking for the crew—mountains of mashed potatoes with craters full of butter, baked beans swimming in pork drippings, chickens who'd lost their heads early that morning, steaks, roasts—often venison from last fall's hunt, chops, ham, whatever vegetables the gardens were yielding just then, and every kind of pickle and jam. And desserts—fresh fruit, pies of every kind, cakes, and cookies. Rarely, ice cream, made that morning. August was the best month, because the corn was ready and the peaches were ripe.

After dinner, he always just wanted to curl up and sleep the rest of the day away, and dream of home. Seven hours of muscle-straining labor could tire a boy out. But the other boys and the men weren't sleepy sissies wanting their mamas, so he wasn't going to be one, either. Any tears were shed soundlessly into his pillow at night.

Greg remembered telling a group of high school boys from someplace in the western part of the state about his boyhood summers; they, too, had worked on harvest crews. One of the boys asked him, "Was there every any—you know—trouble with the men on the haying crews when you were a boy?" Maybe the kid's English teacher had assigned the novel, <u>Of Mice and Men</u>, or maybe he had been a victim.

Greg replied to the awkward question: "If there ever was a pervert on any of the crews I worked with, he was either too tired to bother little boys, or the other men kept a close eye on him. No man ever made a pass at me."

By late August, they were moving from the fields of eastern North Dakota into those of northwestern Minnesota and it was time to go back home and back to school, working at the livery stable after school, and hoping there'd be time for a good gallop down the road.

The nearby farmers kept their horses in their own barns, but the townies rented stalls at the livery stable. The Lutheran minister and the Catholic priest and the doctor all kept their horses and their traps at the livery, and many of the better-off residents also used Greg's dad's business. Those who kept horses mostly to show off how rich they were, but didn't often ride them, encouraged Greg to exercise their stock for them. It never occurred to them to pay him, and he never thought to ask for payment. He loved horses, loved to groom them, talk to them, ride them out into the countryside that smelled so much better than town.

1917
Excited about coming back home after his third harvesting summer, he wasn't prepared for the changes. His dad was drinking again. The new horseless carriages that everyone had scoffed at when one first appeared in town, causing the preacher's horse to shy and dump his rider in the watering trough, were becoming popular, and horses were no longer the main form of transport. The livery stable was history, and that faraway war was coming close to home, taking young men from their family farms and sending them off to fight. Some didn't come home.

Greg assumed Dan was taking him home, to the house in Fargo. No, that wasn't right; that house wasn't theirs anymore. He and Floy had a house in California. So where was she? Maybe she was waiting for him at a hotel. Maybe they would be going back home together. Danny drove to a place with a sign that said Bethany Homes. It looked a bit like a hotel, but Greg could read, and he'd been here before, visiting an old friend. Why were they stopping at a nursing home?

Paul was there—Floy's brother's boy. He invited Greg into a small sitting area, and he talked—slowly and carefully repeating the same things over and over: Alzheimers. Memory loss. Forgetfulness. Unsafe driving. Doctor's care. Medication. Safe place to stay. Family will come to see you.

Paul introduced him to a doctor; Dr. Mazur was his name. The nurse with him was Mrs. Halvorson. Greg knew remembering names was important. The doctor repeated the same things Paul had said. Then they accompanied him to an elevator and led him to a clean but rather bleak bedroom. Mrs. Halvorson said she'd show him around the place. The doctor left. Paul left. Floy wasn't there.

As Mrs. Halvorson showed him around the building, Greg saw some people, reading or watching TV, who smiled at him. Others lolled in wheelchairs, obviously asleep. Mrs. Halvorson took him to the dining room and stayed to have supper with him. The people at the table with him seemed a bit unaware of him or their surroundings, and a couple of them had really dreadful table manners. His mother had always told him that you could tell nice people by nice table manners. Greg wasn't sure he wanted to make many friends here.

September 1987–
September 1988
Nursing Home: First Year

"Memories…a sound, a smell, a word resurrects them."
—Sandra West Prowell

2

CHATTING

Greg liked chatting with Mrs. Halvorson, the nice receptionist here. She listened, and she seemed really interested and she asked good questions. Greg walked over to her desk in the mail lounge, near the front door. She was looking over the menus for the week, so he asked what was planned for lunch.

"There's pork chops and applesauce, with mashed potatoes, green beans, and salad. And apple pie for dessert!" Mrs. Halvorson made the last item sound like a really special treat, so she was a bit taken aback when Greg scowled and asked if they put spices in the apple pie.

She admitted that she wasn't sure, but sounded as if she assumed they did. "Would you find out for me, please?" Greg requested.

A few minutes later, she came over to where he was sitting in front of the TV, not really watching, just brooding. "Greg, I asked about the apple pie—spices, you know. And the cook says they just put sugar and a bit of arrowroot and butter in with the apples. No cinnamon or anything like that."

Greg's face lit up with a beauteous smile. "Thank you! I'll really enjoy lunch, especially the dessert."

"Excuse me asking, Greg, but I thought you would be disappointed that there *weren't* any spices. Is there a story behind that?" the receptionist asked.

Greg laughed and told her the tale. During the first couple years of his marriage with Floy, she occasionally made apple pies—with both cinnamon and nutmeg. He ate the desserts and pretended to enjoy them, but whenever there was a second choice, he always opted for the alternative. Floy finally asked if there was something wrong with her apple pie, and that's when he admitted that he didn't like cinnamon and nutmeg—he really couldn't stand either one. And would she please leave them out in future?

Greg's beloved wife had a stubborn streak, and her feelings had been hurt, he could tell. She did not make another apple pie, with or without spices, for nearly three years. She finally relented when he brought home a half bushel of apples. She made a spiceless apple pie for him, and a fat, bubbly, spicy apple dumpling for herself. Greg had enjoyed unadulterated apple pie ever since.

"I'm glad there isn't going to be another tug of wills ending in a pieless future for me," he said with a sheepish grin.

Larry had just walked in the door, so he joined them, and the three of them started talking about Thanksgiving plans. Mrs. Halvorson said they were getting 25 turkeys from a farm east of Fargo. Greg told her, "I tried raising turkeys once. Now the whole saga seems amusing," and he revealed the whole tale.

Raising turkeys seemed like a good idea at the time. Greg had thought about bison, but turkeys eat less, take up less room, and don't require massive fencing. He had known enough not to get just-hatched turkeys: they need temperature-controlled housing, they need to be weighed individually every day and sometimes force-fed, and they eliminate incredible amounts of foully reeking guano.

Greg got a good deal on five hundred young adult turkeys that just needed fattening up. They grew. The fall was mild, so they were neither too warm nor too cold, and it was too early for storms.

The butcher was scheduled to do half the flock a couple weeks before Thanksgiving, the other half just before Christmas. Greg waited and watched them get fat and planned what to do with the nice profit.

Mrs. Halvorson asked, "Aren't turkeys rather stupid?"

"Well," Greg replied, "Wild turkeys are canny birds. They can hide in trees or on the ground so well that a hunter within a couple feet will not see them. And they can whisper themselves out of danger's way. They can sense a storm coming and take cover. They don't stand around socializing or squabbling with one another and lining up like the Redcoats did during Revolutionary War times, waiting to get shot.

"Domestication, however, has made turkeys one of the all-time idiots of the animal kingdom. I didn't know that at the time. I learned the hard way."

He would never forget the incredible, awful day, two days before the butcher was due, less than a week before he would have made a comfortable profit on each bird. It rained. Not a deluge with howling winds and fireworks in the sky, just a nice, steady rain.

Every last one of the five hundred big, fat, almost ready for the table turkeys lifted its brainless head to the sky and—drowned. They didn't drown in sudden pools of water; their pen was well-drained. Their feet barely got wet. They drowned while ingesting the falling raindrops.

"Chickens," Greg added, "are not noted for intelligence, but even a chicken has the wit to get out of the rain."

Mrs. Halvorson looked a bit dubious. "Greg, is that really a true story?"

"Would I lie to you?" Greg said, looking very earnest.

Mrs. Halvorson asked Larry if his dad really had raised turkeys. Larry glanced at his dad, and with a grin, replied, "Yup. They swallowed buckets of falling rain and drowned."

"You're kidding me!"

"No, and it wasn't funny at the time, but it sure makes a great story now, doesn't it, Dad?"

After Larry had left, Mrs. Halvorson asked Greg if he was expecting friends to visit. He told her that his long-time friend Mike might come.

When he first met Mike, Greg recalled, no one in Fargo or anywhere else in the world had heard of a man called Hitler, or ever seen his picture. So it didn't matter that Mike looked like a happy, pudgy, Adolf Hitler, complete with a mustache that resembled a much-used toothbrush and straight, dark hair that fell over his forehead like a roofing tile. Years later, when Hitler's face, name, and hysteria-inducing, mob inciting voice had become frighteningly familiar, Mike shaved the mustache, had his hair cut military short, and was careful never to scowl. Mike's voice was a rumbly bass, and no one remembered that Mike had ever looked like anyone but himself.

He told Mrs. Halvorson about the time he and Mike came home on the train together. He didn't remember the train ride, but he remembered why they couldn't drive home.

1943

After a week of morning temperatures more than 30 degrees below zero, mornings so still they could hear the ice crackle and settle, mornings of sunlight trying to push faintly through the fog of snow, mornings so cold his eyebrows froze into spikes of ice—after that week, a February thaw turned the snow-plowed drifts lining the road-

sides into walls of ice that oozed water onto the roads, water that froze again into patches of black ice.

Mike and he had just topped a hill when they hit one of those patches, a long one, an ice slide clear to the bottom of the hill. He'd barely tapped the brakes, but even that was too much. Instantly, the car spun and kept spinning, round and round like some of the scarier carnival rides, until it was stopped abruptly by a snow bank at the roadside. Mike and he were breathing heavily and checking out fingers, toes, arms, legs, shoulders—nothing broken. For a moment, they thought they could drive on, even more slowly than before.

Maybe they heard something. Maybe they just thought it was too much to hope that they would emerge unscathed. They both looked up, to see the huge truck bearing down on them, wheels locked, spinning seemingly slowly, but inexorably, at them, into them.

Greg remembered how he had regretted the death of that car. And how he and Mike, neither very religious, got down on their knees in the snow, with the truck driver, to give thanks. He also remembered that Floy, who was shaken, but practical, needed assurance that the car had been insured—and that he and Mike were okay. Mariette, Mike's wife, had hysterics.

Thinking of Mariette, Greg smiled. She was a big woman, fond of food, generous to friends and not-friends, always beautifully dressed and beautifully groomed. Greg and Floy loved her name and always called her Mariette. Mike called her Babe—always. Mariette and Floy were unlikely, but inevitable friends. Courted by their husbands during and after college, married about the same time, and obliged to spend time together so Mike and Greg could continue to build their friendship, they shared childhoods of never enough food or money for extras, but they did not share their habits of dealing with those memories.

Floy considered cooking a duty, not a pleasure. She prepared simple meals, rarely invited friends for dinner, required Clean Plate Club rules of her kids, never suggested going out for dinner. Her refrigerator and cupboards were stocked with one week's groceries. She did not have and did not want a separate freezer. Floy ate sparingly and, except for pregnancies, never weighed more—or less—than 112 pounds. Greg loved every inexpensively but neatly dressed ounce.

From conversations with Mike and Floy and from his own observations, Greg knew a lot about Mariette. She loved to cook, but did so rarely, and then only an elaborate feast for at least six guests. Her kids fixed their own peanut butter and jelly sandwiches and disappeared before guests arrived. Mostly, she and Mike ate out, at restaurants or friends' homes. Her refrigerator, separate freezer, and cupboards, both at the house in town and the cottage at Detroit Lake, were stuffed with enough food to feed her own family and several others for months. Most of it was never used. Twice a year, Mariette cleaned out her refrigerator, freezer, and cupboards and donated the contents to charity. She did enjoy shopping—for food she would never eat, for clothes, for gifts for friends. And she loved to eat elsewhere than her own home.

Mariette dieted constantly, by skipping breakfast, meeting friends for lunch ("just a little salad please," topped off with sundaes, éclairs, pie, cake, and sundry other desserts.) During the week while Mike was on the road, she shopped, played bridge, and nibbled her way though nuts, chocolates, and potato chips the rest of the day. When Mike got home for the weekend, or was home for the whole summer, they went out for dinner. Mike loved every one of his wife's beautifully groomed, elegantly dressed 225 pounds.

Floy had told Greg that she did not understand Mariette's addiction to clothes shopping. As he knew, Floy usually bought the first thing she tried on, and she tried things on only twice a year. Mariette had weekly manicures and hair appointments, and—her one vanity—so did Floy, who had been brought up, she had told Greg more than once, that a lady can be judged by really good shoes, really good gloves, and really good grooming.

Greg remembered playing cards with Babe and Mike, going to the same parties, staying at each other's summer places, and never running out of conversation. They talked about their children—Mike and Babe had five: a boy and girl older than Larry, a boy Judie's age, a boy a bit older than Jeannie, and a menopause baby, spoiled by everyone, who surprised everyone by not winding up in prison.

He wasn't sure he should tell this, but he did: the boy Judie's age was her date for the junior prom, arranged by both mothers. Bob had never dated, never did, in fact, and he and Floy wondered a bit about him. They were sorry for his parents when the boy turned out to be queer. He never mentioned it to Mike.

Greg explained to Mrs. Hal (he wasn't sure if her name was Hanson or Haliburton or Halvorson, so he had started calling her Mrs. Hal, which seemed to amuse her) that he and Mike had both intended to be teachers, but the scarcity of openings and the inadequate salaries turned them to other careers. They both spent their days in schools, but the services they provided had nothing to do with books. Mike was the area representative for a company that produced cleaning materials and preservatives for classroom, hall, and gymnasium floors and walls. Greg's company manufactured class rings, athletic medals and trophies, and graduation announcements.

Greg remembered that he and Mike had coined the word "carpool" long before it came into common usage. They called on most of the same schools, so during the war, to save precious gas coupons, they traveled together, using his car one week, Mike's the next. They talked a lot, while driving and while staying in small town hotels during the week. Both were concerned about the way school consolidation was changing the state's small towns. Many of their schools graduated only a few students a year—and none some years. Already, some of those small schools had closed their doors and the kids who would never graduate from them were bused long miles from their home-towns, in which they would not live as adults.

Economically, Greg thought, perhaps school consolidation made sense, but small towns were dying, and as far as he and Mike were concerned, the quality of education was not improved. They both knew many bright, prosperous young people who had come from one-room schoolhouses whose spinster teachers taught reading, writing, and 'rithmetic to maybe 15 or 20 kids, first grade through eighth.

Curly, a long-time friend of Larry's, had finished the eighth grade at one of those now defunct one-room schoolhouses, near Valley City. And then he had apprenticed to a stone mason. Curly was an artist with stone. His fire-places, patios, churches, museums, and a very rare few homes could be found all over the state.

Curly was here with Larry to take Greg out for lunch. They had a favorite watering hole with an unpretentious name, "The Steak House."

Occasionally women showed up there for lunch, but it was really a man's place. Oak floors, spotlessly clean but bare of rugs. A long, glossy-shiny bar—teak, maybe—you could see your reflection in it. An honest-to-good-ness brass rail and spittoons, although these days gentlemen didn't spit. The wall behind the bar was a solid array of bottles of every size, shape, and color—one long, thin, mantis-green one full of some liqueur he'd never heard of. And no-nonsense booths, oak again.

The menu offered everything from hamburgers and quiche (which, Greg had heard, real men don't eat; he'd never tried it) to the steaks the place was noted for. And fresh, homemade bread, still warm from the oven. They all ordered beer—Hamms on tap.

1960

Greg remembered hiring Curly to redo the fireplace at the lake after the fire that could have, but didn't, burn down the cottage. Curly was delighted—"My first foreign job!"

He spent weeks hunting for the rocks he wanted—they had to be local rocks, not just ordinary local rocks, but rocks that would talk to each other. Greg wanted to watch as the new fireplace grew, but was refused. Curly just said that if Greg didn't like the final result, he would tear it down and start over, but he wouldn't allow anyone to oversee its creation.

Greg had thought the old fireplace adequate—bumpy rocks stuck together with concrete—more concrete than rocks—with a smooth hearth and a plank mantelpiece. The sort of fireplace that did its job, warming the cottage without choking the inhabitants with smoke. The sort of fireplace that no one really noticed.

Curly's fireplace captured the eye of everyone entering the room. Varying shades of light tan rock provided an arresting contrast to the dark log walls. Rugged in outline, but smooth on the surface, each rock almost but not quite touched its neighbor, with just a bit of concrete to outline each shape. It soared to the stone slab mantel echoing the hearth below. Greg was enchanted.

"Greg, dija hear about Ole and Swen and Lena getting lost in the woods and finding a bottle?" "Nope, haven't heard that one." "Well, there they were…"

Greg chuckled to himself: Curly not only created works of art in stone, he was also an incorrigible story teller. He repeated stories only on request—his supply was limitless. Greg's favorites were the Ole, Swen, and Lena stories, told in Curly's very accurate and very funny Norwegian accent. Greg sometimes wondered if Curly's first language had maybe not been English.

"There they were, lost in the woods and getting colder and hungrier by the minute, when Lena finds this bottle, half-buried by tree roots. She yanks it out and starts rubbing it to clean it up, and guess what?"

"What?"

"Out pops a genie and he tells them he will grant each of them a wish, three being the magic number for wishes, doncha know. So Lena closes her eyes and makes a wish—to be safely back home. Poof! Lena's gone. Then Swen closes his eyes and makes a wish—to be safely home with Lena. Poof! Swen's gone. Ole dances from one foot to the other, trying to think of a more exciting wish than just going home. Eureka! He's got it! 'I vish Sven and Lena wuz here with me.'"

◆   ◆   ◆

He was glad Jeannie and Judie were with him; he hoped they had come to take him home. They explained that they had come to visit, and would come as often as they could, but while the doctors were doing tests to determine what was causing the memory lapses, he would have to stay here.

Sometimes he feared that it was not a temporary stay. He wanted to go home. He did not belong in a hospital. There was nothing wrong with his memory, just too much to remember after so many years.

He told Larry the next time he came that he didn't like being in a hospital when he wasn't sick. Larry pointed out that the place was really more like a quite elegant hotel, with comfortable bedrooms, nicely decorated and furnished lounge areas, each with two or three TV sets, an ice cream parlor, and a pleasant dining room. And even a barber shop, where an expert would properly trim his hair, comb-over and all.

The next time his daughters came, he proudly took them on a tour, arriving at the ice cream parlor just as everyone was ready for a treat. It was his favorite place—red and white candy-striped walls, old-fashioned stools along the soda fountain counter, and ice cream cones as good as the Dairy Maid offered. They agreed this was as nice a hotel as they'd ever seen. He didn't ask if it was really a hotel; he did not want to know for sure.

"No, Daddy, we can't stay here with you. We both have to get home to our families and jobs." He remembered. They didn't live in the Fargo house any more. Jeannie was in Minneapolis; Judie was in Michigan someplace. He'd been there once, he thought. His memory had holes in it.

◆   ◆   ◆

Greg wondered if maybe his eyesight was as bad as his memory. He used to talk to his reflection in the mirror, as he shaved, planning the day ahead. He avoided looking in mirrors these days. What looked back at him the last time he did look wasn't him. He stood tall, shoulders back, proud of his six-foot height. That person in the mirror slouched. Greg had the thick, richly black, wavy hair, cornflower blue eyes, and fair, unblemished skin of the true "black Norwegian." Looking back at him was a nearly bald man with a bit of whitish-gray fuzz around the edges, and a long lanky piece from the back wound around the hairless crown of his head. The reflection's eyes were a washed-out gray, and its skin was mottled and pasty. If Greg did say so himself—never out loud—he was a handsome young man. His supposed mirror image was a rather shrunken, dowdy oldster. Why anyone would play silly games, like covering mirrors with ugly pictures, he couldn't imagine.

Come to think of it, though, he did have a little patch with no hair on the crown of his head. He had learned how to do an artful comb-over so it didn't show, but one time when he and a couple of the grandkids were swimming in the lake, his grandson Mark had broadcast to the whole world "Grandpa's bald!" One cannot maintain an artful comb-over while doing the Australian crawl.

He wished Floy were here. Her eyes always reflected the man she married. She should be here. He'd been in hotels before without her, but that was when he was working, and he had retired—hadn't he? And was this really a hotel?

Larry had been evasive when asked where Floy was, muttering something about the house in California. What house in California? Was his son trying to start a fly-by-night business and had he conned his mother into helping? Judie and Jeanne had also said Floy was in California and would come as soon as she sold the house. Greg didn't know anything about a house in California. They'd stayed in a rental condo on the California coast several times during the winter, and had talked about building a house out there, but he didn't think they had actually done that. He wished Floy would come; he had so many questions to ask her.

Maybe Obert would come; his farm was close to Fargo. No, Obert wouldn't come; he had died a couple years ago. Nineteen years older than Greg, he had almost made it to his 100th birthday.

Obert looked like a farmer: big-boned, ham-handed, overalled, walnut-brown tanned from forehead to collar and arms just above the elbow, milk white below the collar, squint wrinkles and laugh lines around eyes that never looked through sunglasses, deep laugh lines around the mouth.

Obert laughed, and made other people laugh and believe that the world was a pretty comic place. His blue eyes, like his mother's, like Greg's, twinkled.

His pre-retirement, pre-nursing home life was not easy, but he had a build-in pair of rose-colored classes. Of his homesteading years in Montana, Obert remembered and talked about the unusual, the interesting, the entertaining—never the hardships of

subzero Montana winters in a sod hut with attendant frostbite and howling bliz-
zards.

After proving his homestead, Obert and his wife Anna returned to northwest Min-
nesota, returned to farming, the only life they ever really wanted. Anna was a strong,
uncomplaining, plain woman—plain until she smiled and her love for her husband,
everyone's child, and baby pigs, cows, chickens, and even geese set her glowing from
within.

As a child, Greg had hardly known his oldest brother. The family was still living
on the farm and Greg hadn't yet started school when Obert went west. He did remem-
ber Obert's return, full of stories and happiness. Hard to believe that he, too, was the
son of that dour, sour father. Maybe because Obert didn't drink.

Greg loved visiting Obert and Anna. Their home was rich with laughter and
horses and love and his favorite foods and kids. His oldest nephews and nieces were
right about his own age. He remembered romping in the hayloft, jumping down onto
hay piles on the barn floor. He remembered climbing haystacks in the fields and,
shouting "Geronimo!" sliding down, feeling the caress of wind on his cheeks. He and
the other kids thought school playground slides were pretty tame after haystacks.

Greg outgrew haystack slides, but he never outgrew his ties to Obert and Anna and
their farm. Until the move to California, he visited often—once a month at least.
Larry often went with him; Floy never allowed him to take Judie.

Maybe it was Larry's eager questions about homesteading and wolves and panning
icy mountain streams for non-existent gold that nudged Obert into writing his autobi-
ography. Maybe it was that after such an active life, he wasn't about to vegetate in a
nursing home, even if he was 97 years old.

**Greg fervently hoped that he, too, would find himself writing his life
story at the age of 97, but if he really was losing his marbles (as a child, he'd
thought that expression was a riot; now it was a terrifying possibility), he
would not choose to live. But who ever can choose? Nowadays, none of those
things that used to take people quickly when it was their time—and even
before their time—seemed to be able to withstand new-fangled medical
interference. Looking around at the human husks lolling in their wheelchairs, he doubted that most of them would choose to be here.**

September 1988–September 1989 Nursing Home: Second Year

"He travels in his mind now."
—Phil Frank & Joe Troise

3

COME TO VISIT

He needed his wife. He needed to talk to her.

Greg talked to anyone who would listen, and the nurses were good listeners, especially Mrs. Hal. And when the kids visited, they still seemed to enjoy his stories. Roger, a new friend, a young man who had visited often and stayed for several hours each time, went for walks with him, and had listened well at first.

They were sitting in one of the lounges. Roger asked, "Did your mother work?"

"Oh, yes, she worked—dawn to dusk every day."

"What did she do?"

"Well, Mondays she did the laundry."

"A lot of women do laundry on Mondays, and other days as well, but they still work," Roger remarked.

"You are very young, aren't you? I know that a lot of women now can throw a load of laundry in a washing machine when they get up, toss it in the dryer as soon as they've brushed their teeth, sort it while they're munching a quickie breakfast and downing a cup of coffee, and dash off to the office.

"When I was a boy, laundry was all day. After cooking breakfast for all of us, Mother would fire up the clothes boiler, stir in the soap when the water was hot, drop in the sheets and other whites, and stir it all with a wooden paddle. Handkerchiefs were boiling in a pot on the stove. Then she'd haul out the wringer—a hand cranked contraption with rollers that each wet piece of laundry had to be guided through with one hand while cranking with the other. Unless a child not yet old enough for school could do the cranking. For a while, that was me.

"That load went into a rinse tub before getting cranked through the wringer again. Then a light-colored load was started, and finally the dark work clothes. The washing would take all morning."

Greg could remember how hot and steamy the kitchen got, steam rising to the ceiling to cool into globules that dripped down into the bubbling cauldron of clothes and onto his mother's shoulders and hair—its usual tidy bun losing tendrils that she futilely tried pushing back into submission with a damp hand.

Roger was looking fidgety, but he had asked, so Greg continued, with fewer details. "After she prepared lunch for those of us who came home for it, Mother took the basket of wet clothes outside and pegged each piece on the clothesline. While they dried in the wind and sun, she started chopping and peeling, getting started on supper. Then she unpegged each dry piece of laundry, sorted and folded and put the things that needed ironing—including sheets—in the ironing basket, ready for Tuesday, ironing day. Would you like me to continue?" Greg was getting a bit irritated at the obvious boredom of this young man.

"No, I get the idea. So your mother didn't have a job?"

Exasperated, Greg replied, "My mother's job, which ate up far more than forty hours a week, and which she did superbly, was to feed, clothe, care for, and clean up after her husband and seven children. She did that her entire life. If she was lucky, she might get an occasional 'thank you.' She did not get a paycheck.

"Don't you have someplace to go, young man? I'm going to have a nap," Greg almost snarled as he got up and walked over to Mrs. Hal, at her desk.

He asked her why that guy was always hanging around. "If they think I need a baby-sitter, could you ask them to get someone who doesn't think he knows it all?"

Mrs. Hal suggested that they get a cup of coffee and chat for a bit. "I remember my grandmother talking about raising a family. She'd have been about your mother's age. She told us how each child had chores to do after school and on weekends. I know you helped your dad at the livery stable. What did you kids do for fun?"

Mollified, Greg smiled. "We were all busy, adults and kids, but not frantic busy like so many people now. It was a kind of slow and easy busy. None of us went far from home very often, because mostly we had to walk wherever we were going. Adults walked briskly; kids dawdled. You notice a lot more when you're walking. We watched the ungreening of the trees as they put on their fall wardrobes of bright colors. How does that poem go—'the yellow and the purple and the crimson...and the scarlet of the maples can shake me like the cry of bugles going by.' Whoever wrote that wasn't whizzing by in a car.

"As kids we had chores, but we also had fun. We played tag and hide-and-seek and kick-the-can and Red Rover. We had disorganized and unsponsored football, basketball, hockey, and baseball games. We had snowball fights. We roller skated and ice skated. We played in, around, and on top of haystacks. We had time to spend an hour watching an anthill or, lying on our backs on the ground, picking out the pictures in the ever-changing clouds. We didn't have to dash home from school, change clothes, and be driven off to piano or dancing lessons, or some other loathsome activity designed to keep kids out of their parents' hair. And our mothers were always home for us."

◆　　　◆　　　◆

Roger didn't come back, but there was another one, Karl, he said his name was. Greg noticed that any visitor who seemed to get bored by his stories didn't return, but was always replaced by a new one, one who seemed enthralled, at least for a while. But it was hard to remember who had heard which stories. Where was Floy? She had always helped make conversation with people.

He asked his nice nurse, Mrs. Hal, where his wife was. (He wasn't always sure if her name was Hanson or something similar, so he called her Mrs. Hal, which seemed to amuse her.) She said Floy was on her way. Greg was eager to see his wife again; it had been a long time. He couldn't remember how long, but he didn't think she had been here all winter, and he knew she wasn't here for Christmas. This gray-haired lady walking toward him with a pained smile on her face—did he know her? When she said, "Hello, dear," he wanted to escape. No! He did not know this woman! But the more she talked, the more familiar the voice sounded. And the eyes, even behind those glasses—he knew those eyes. But she was old. Maybe he was old, too. Maybe the mirror had not lied.

She said she had to leave for a while, but would be back. She hugged him and kissed him, a rather dry, quick kiss. He remembered a better one.

1967
Everyone that Christmas had to have a turn taking pictures with the new home movie camera. There were pictures of Larry and his wife Susie smooching it up under the mistletoe, and Judie and Neil lost to the outside world, and Jeannie and Chris, a bit self conscious, and then he and Floy showed them how it should be done. The kids looked a bit stunned—their parents necking? After thirty-five years of marriage, kissing Floy still made his toes curl.

He wished Floy would visit more often; Larry seemed to come more frequently than she did. He'd heard one of the spy-companions talking to Larry—as if Greg wasn't there or was deaf or stupid: "I've met your two sisters; nice ladies. Does your dad have any sisters? He's only mentioned a brother, and none of his family have been here to see him."

He had had three sisters, one never seen, spoken to or about since their parents' fiftieth anniversary party; the other two gone, their deaths half a century apart. Greg didn't really remember Mabel. She had died when he was only six. Influenza had hit the Midwest—not the world-wide pandemic in the middle of that innocence-killing war, but a devastating epidemic nonetheless, although big-city newspapers ignored it. Almost everyone in town lost someone. It was his big sister Mabel that Greg's family lost, leaving a grieving husband who could not cope with his infant daughter, or much of anything else. Mabel died alone except for her infant daughter. Her husband was in town on some real or imagined errand, figuring she'd get over her cold soon and there was no need for the doctor. There was no money for doctors.

Greg had heard those details from his big sister Hylda, his practical, do-for-others sister who had taken a pony cart out to bring baby Hazel home. Hylda had just started high school, taking a secretarial course. She and Louis were also courting, but any wedding would have to wait, she announced, until Hazel grew up.

Like everyone else in the family, Hylda was a Lutheran, but she never was the usual kind of Lutheran Greg had grown up with. He knew ministers and sermons and churches had changed since he was young. The Presbyterians that his kids had rejected as soon as they could no longer preached hellfire and damnation with lots of brimstone, and the Lutheran message he had turned his back on had brightened up.

But he remembered the old version: big on the ten "Thou shalt nots," almost ignoring the two that Christ had said were the most important of all, and adding another bunch even more important than the first ten. He assumed the minister rotated his sermons to cover them all, over and over: no card games, no alcohol, no dancing, no smoking, no cussing, no fraternizing with non-Lutherans (except as business required)—they're all going to hell and they'll drag you with them, work hard six days and spend the seventh in church and reading the Bible.

After he left home, Greg went inside churches only for funerals and weddings. But he was aware that "Love thy neighbor" and "Love thy God" had pretty much replaced the old commandments. So he guessed it was okay with the church now to love non-Lutherans. He did. Hylda had figured that out long before the church did.

He didn't know if drinking, smoking, card-playing, and dancing were allowed yet; he didn't care. He unrepentantly indulged in all four—in moderation.

Hylda was not the dour, sour non-church-going alcoholic kind of Lutheran their dad seemed to be; not the slightly vague, husband-knows-best doormat kind of Lutheran wife Greg sometimes thought his mother was. Hylda was more like Obert, fun-loving, optimistic, cheerful, taking care of every waif dog or cat or duck or child she could find. She was a regular church-goer, but her relationship with God wasn't just a Sunday thing; she seemed to share frequent daily conversations with Him, like two housewives chatting over coffee and cookies.

Hylda wasn't pretty like Rosella. Hylda was stocky, partly because she was a superb cook and she loved to eat. Her legs were covered with wrinkly lisle stockings and skirts that stopped at mid-calf. Her feet were stuffed into old-lady shoes from the time she was a teen. Her mousy hair was always pulled back into a no-nonsense, no-fuss bun at the back of her head. Her lively blue eyes hid behind unattractive glasses. But Hylda glowed from within, and to everyone who knew her, she was beautiful.

December at Hylda's was a sugar-fest: rosettes and krumkaka and pfeffersneuse and other Christmas goodies were always flaunting themselves, tempting every visitor to forget the diet and start believing an additional five pounds wouldn't matter.

Greg visited her in the hospital a week before the cancer killed her, hoping to be able to cheer her and pray with her. He was not really surprised when Hylda turned the tables on him—she consoled and cheered him. She was not in pain, she said, and she had tried to live her life so God would be pleased with her when she joined Him. She was eagerly waiting for that moment. Greg always enjoyed visiting with her; he knew God had, too; Hylda was good company.

Karl was here again. He said something about keeping Greg company until his wife Floy, his son Larry, and his daughters, Judie and Jeannie could visit. Why was he making such a point of telling him their names? He knew the names of his dear family! And why were they visiting him here, in this hotel? They all lived in the big white house on First Street, didn't they? Greg was sure he remembered that.

The young man—his name was Karl; he must try to remember that—was talking about the college he went to. Greg went to college. Or he used to. It was all so confusing, the now and the then. Remembering college helped him believe he was not losing his mind.

1923–25

After Greg graduated from high school, he had escaped the dead end of the small town. There was a teachers' college in Valley City, and one of his teachers had a friend who owned a farm outside of town. He could board there, helping out around the farm while taking classes. In those days, teaching credentials required only two years of college, and he could get by on little money for that short a time. His mother had given him a precious going away present—half of his wages from the previous summer's hayfields. He'd always given her all his earnings, knowing that money was very tight.

Greg was delighted to find that the kind of help needed by the family he boarded with was taking care of the horses. In addition to their own riding horses, the family had two pairs of draft horses. They were still doing most of their farming the old way, with horse-drawn plows, drags, and wagons, and they rode their horses into town. They had an automobile, but it had a habit of breaking down on the way to town.

Karl was still talking about college. Greg interrupted him—he'd been to college, too.

He remembered Miss Sweeney, who taught speech and coached the debate team, and taught him to breathe properly while giving a speech: she told him to tighten his abdominal muscles and take deep breaths. To check that indeed the muscles were tight, she punched him, not gently, in the solar plexus.

Greg punched Ken—or was his name Karl?—to demonstrate, and suddenly he was surrounded by white coats and someone stuck a needle in his arm. Did they think he was trying to hurt someone? He had never hit anyone who hadn't hit him first and wasn't at least his size. He fell asleep, dreaming about college.

He dreamed about a girlfriend. Was her name Floy? No, she came later. That girl was May or Maisie or something. She was a student in one of his classes, boarding with a family at a farm a couple miles from his temporary home, and they began a tentative courtship. To visit her, Greg borrowed one of the horses and rode across the fields for occasional evenings of stiffly sitting in the neighbors' parlor or, in good weather, rocking with the girl on the porch glider.

One evening he set out for a visit despite warnings of an impending snowstorm, figuring he would be back safe before it got bad. But he stayed longer than he had planned, and by the time he started back, the snow was coming down hard, and the wind was blowing it in every direction. Drifts were piling up. He could not see the lights of his farmhouse, and after he'd gone a short distance, he couldn't see the lights of the farm he'd just left, either.

He knew midwestern blizzards were nothing to mess with. Farm families, and the wiser ones in towns, tied a long length of clothesline to the back doorknob, long enough to loop around the waist of a person who had to get to the barn to tend the livestock or a townie who might have to get to a neighbor's for help. Tragedies happened to the careless. A neighbor boy had let his six-year-old sister go with him to the barn during one such storm. Previous winters had been mild, so there was no lifeline. The boy made it to the barn, but the wind whipped the child from his handclasp. They found her six weeks later, when the snow melted, 100 yards from the house.

Greg knew he was in trouble. He could ride in circles in the snow until the horse fell, exhausted. And no one would find them until it was too late. There was no choice but to trust his horse to find the way home. People had let him down at times, but no horse ever had. A horse would always do what was expected, if it was trained properly, and if its rider knew how to ask. Greg loosed his hold on the reins, giving the horse its head, and they floundered on through the storm. He lost the feeling in his feet and his hands, but he kept his light hold on the reins and his seat in the saddle. When they finally saw lights in the near distance, the horse picked up the pace—he was home. Greg had to be lifted off his back.

He must have dozed off. Kurt—was that his name? Greg was having trouble remembering new names—was asking, "Were you a teacher, then?" That hadn't been in his dream, but whatever was had gone.

4

COLLEGE, COURTSHIP, AND CHILDREN

   Greg remembered the two years of teaching in small high schools that did not always have a graduating class every year. He loved the students, he enjoyed the simple social life with his colleagues, he respected the administrators and their staff people. In fact, he had decided that with another two years of college, he, too, would have the necessary credentials to become a principal and superintendent. He had carefully saved enough money to do that.

   This time he would get involved in real college life, adding fun and friendship to classes, work, and study. He went to fraternity rushes, not sure that scene was right for him, but not ready to dismiss it without checking it out. At one party, he met Mike, who advised Greg to join a fraternity—not necessarily ATO, although in Mike's opinion it was the best.

   Mike told Greg that fraternities were the best introduction to people who could open professional doors after graduation. And a fraternity house was the cheapest place to live, the best place to meet girls, and a great place to drink with friends. Greg avoided the drinking pretty much—he'd seen enough of those problems in his father—but he pledged ATO and never regretted it.

   The ATO house was, indeed, a great place to meet girls. At a party in the spring, Greg delightedly watched an adorable flapper dancing on one of the tables. He quietly asked for an introduction. Floy was also a third year education major—at the tender age of 18. They shared several classes, as well as parties, picnics, and occasionally the pictures. Floy was hooked on the weekly installments of "The Perils of Pauline."

   Every Saturday afternoon, they sat holding hands, watching as Pauline was tied to railroad tracks by the villain, rescued by the hero, and then dangled from a rope over a cliff, not to be rescued from that peril until the next Saturday, when new perils awaited.

Greg loved Floy's keen mind, her glee at watching Pauline get herself in trouble, her dancing legs, her cap of dark hair, her somber eyes, her quick smile. He loved her—everything about her. They talked about marriage, but it would have to wait until they both had jobs.

"So you were a teacher?" That young man again, interrupting his thoughts. Greg wished Ken?—his name didn't matter—would go away and let him bask in his memories. Maybe he was some kind of spy. He was always there, it seemed. But why would anyone keep watching him? He wasn't going anyplace. He enjoyed taking walks when someone was with him—preferably one of his children—but he was afraid to go out of the building by himself. He wasn't sure he could find his way back if he walked by himself. And he would never risk crossing a street alone—too many cars, going too fast. He had always preferred small towns with little traffic. But he did like to drive—he'd always driven a lot.

1929–32

Every Saturday morning, Greg drove his battered but dependable Model T from Arena, the small, dusty, poverty-locked town where he was the high school principal, where his best friend and landlord was the janitor. His destination initially was tiny Parshall, and later slightly larger Valley City, where Floy taught in other high schools, where most of the boys were both older and bigger than she, and where her 9-month salary was $1200. They spent time sipping coffee in the towns' dingy cafés, going for walks, and returning to the cafés for the dinner special, which was cheap, carefully splitting the bill because Floy insisted. At eight o'clock, they snuck a kiss and Greg got back in the Model T and drove back to Arena.

The drive took him past the small, dying towns of North Dakota and the miles and miles of parched, barren, once-lush fields between them. Yet green buds of hope appeared from the tiny branches of saplings planted on the western edges of farms—to hold the earth, to shelter it from the dust storms and the winter blizzards.

Greg told his companion about one year when a band of men from who knows where, put to work by the CCC, planted 100 saplings, a few oak, a few elm, mostly evergreens, in a mile-long row on the west side of the NDAC campus, on the edge of town. The bankers and lawyers and shopkeepers guffawed in disdain—planted in November, those sad, spindly sticks would never survive the harsh winter. Those who lived and loved and understood the earth waited. Years later, when that faraway war started, the war that came too close to home and changed lives forever, ninety-seven of those trees proudly buffered the city, holding in the soil, holding back the wind with their lofty branches.

His blond daughter—Jeannie was her name—had taken him for a drive out that way a few days ago. The trees still stood sentinel, protecting the city, holding the storms at bay. He could ask that young man who visited every day to drive out there again. No, that young man had stopped coming. But there was another spy. Actually, Shirley was okay. She was a fat, friendly woman who seemed to have nothing better to do than drive him to the river for lovely long walks along the river bank and then to the Dairy Maid ice cream store which had the best sugar cones piled high with their homemade vanilla ice cream. And she talked with him and listened to his memories. "You're married, aren't you? I think I've seen your wife."

1932

The day after April Fool's—they laughed about that for years—Greg drove to Valley City, Floy got in the car, they drove to Fargo to pick up her mother, her sister Hope, and Hope's husband Alex, and drove to Lake Park, where they were married. Only one other person was included—Greg's mother. Back to Fargo to return Hope and Alex to their home, and the newlyweds, with Greg's new mother-in-law, boarded the train to Minneapolis for their honeymoon weekend. Floy's mother was necessary—female teachers could not be married women, so a chaperone was needed if an unmarried lady were to travel with a man. Someone might see them.

They had to keep up the charade until the end of the school year. More Saturdays in Valley City; long lonely days between. Floy was going to resign at the end of the school year anyway, but by June the cat had to come out of the bag—she was pregnant.

"You have children, don't you? Didn't I hear that your son and his wife are coming to take you out this afternoon?" Shirley again, but the interruption was okay; she sounded really interested.

February 1933

He had a son! Greg had never thought much about babies, except that when Hylda brought Mabel's motherless baby home, he'd abruptly become just another kid to feed and send to school and do chores. As the baby of the family for six years, he had enjoyed being cuddled and cherished. His mother had still tried, but that baby took up a lot of time that once had been his.

But this was his son, his first born, his child to teach and protect and hone into manhood. So tiny. Those feet! Human feet, he felt, were possibly the least attractive part of human anatomy, but these baby feet were adorable. Perfectly formed, soft as satin, and they wiggled. Soft baby hands, too, already grasping and waving.

Those hands weren't so cute clenched in Larry's lap while the police asked him about the flaming curtains in the empty house across the street from the school. Larry was only eight, and after warning about the dangers of playing with matches and saying boys will be boys, the law left. Greg could not let it go at that. His blood ran cold at the thought of what might have happened: his son a charred corpse in a burned-out house.

He wanted to embrace his son and never let him go. The prank could not go unpunished. Those baby hands had been perverted. Greg's father had used a razor strap on him when he sinned, and Greg knew no other way of expressing his shame and disappointment—and love.

Larry's hands on a football, basketball, or baseball were magic. Greg's childhood had had little time for sports, so he reveled in his son's athletic skills, only wishing the boy cared half as much for his studies.

When he got to college, Larry seemed to be applying himself. Not with distinction, but with adequacy. But then those itchy hands led to a week's suspension. He and some friends had, with their bare hands, demolished a plywood barrier intended to prevent traffic through the underground heat tunnels from the men's dorm to the women's. The boys were caught, because the roommate of the girl they were visiting at 2 a.m.—the girl Larry later married—was not pleased to see them. She screamed and woke up the housemother.

When Larry arrived home for his week's banishment, Greg thought about disowning him, refusing to continue paying his tuition, making him get a job. But he had not raised a son to put him through the struggles he himself had endured. And deep down, he wasn't sure that he wouldn't have been part of a similar caper if he had had the opportunity when he was nineteen.

Greg got his revenge when Larry's first son, Mark, was born. Looking at Larry's face when he held his newborn, Greg could see the same wonder, the same hopes and fears he had felt as a new father.

Shirley interrupted his thoughts again: "I enjoyed meeting your older daughter. Nice of her to come all this way to see you."

1934

Judie wasn't planned. If Floy and he had planned when to have a second child, it would not have been when Larry was still in diapers, when they were barely able to pay the rent on the ramshackle one-bedroom house, when Floy would be waddling in the advanced stages of pregnancy through the hottest summer on record.

If he hadn't taken Judie for her pre-school doctor's checkup, he would never have met the fraternity brother to whom he had loaned money years before. And he would never have been offered the mortgaged farm in payment of that debt. And he would never have had the pure joy of spending Saturdays with his son and daughter, calling the horses in from the pasture, currying them, saddling them up, and riding for hours with the clean wind in their faces. If Judie came today, maybe they could drive out to the farm and go for a ride. The last time they had a ride together seemed longer ago than just last weekend.

Yes, it was wonderful to see Judie. But something was wrong with his brain. Every time Judie came, he had to ask someone if that really was his daughter. The Judie of now had laugh lines and crows' feet. When she sat down and hugged him and started talking, he remembered the now, but before he heard her voice, he expected to see a pig-tailed child with glasses, in riding boots, or a young bride in her wedding gown.

1956

If only his mother could have seen him in full formal morning dress, top hat and all, looking like the polished, urbane, man-of-the-world he had become. Almost. Part of him was forever the innocent, naïve, dirt-poor farm boy from northwestern Minnesota.

Judie's wedding. He and Floy and wide-eyed thirteen-year-old Jeannie had sailed with the bride-to-be from Montreal to Southampton; left Judie in the care of her impending husband and father-in-law while the banns were called in the local church; and set off on a three-week exploration of a bit of France and a lot of the British Isles.

He and Floy had been married nearly 25 years and this second honeymoon had everything the first one hadn't—time for loving, eating, dancing, and being entertained on board the ship, and time for poking in charming little shops in quaint little villages as well as grand old cities.

All the sight-seeing in England and a bit of the continent lived up to the guidebooks, but the one place that would stay in his mind forever was a little English farm near where the tour bus temporarily broke down. The house was like his birth home, with a kitchen that was the everything-else room, complete with a stone sink and a trap bucket under the drain; a parlor, for the pastor's rare visits and funeral afters; three bedrooms, each with a double bed: one room for the boys, one for the girls, one for the parents and the newest baby. The privy was outside the back door, at the end of the small garden. There was running water—at the barn pump—that was carried to the house in buckets as needed.

The little cottage in St. Andrews that Judie and that man would be living in at least had indoor plumbing. Actually, it was a charming place. But the more he saw of the bridegroom, the less charming he found him. Too late. The Yorkshire newspapers were full of pictures and stories about the Americans who had come 5,000 miles for their daughter's wedding to a local boy. Sailing for home the day after the wedding, leaving Judie alone with that man and too far away to come home, he worried.

Later—a lot later, he thought; years later, he thought—when Judie phoned to say she and Neil were divorcing, Floy said it for both of them: "It's about time." And later than that, when Judie said that she and her friend Al were going to marry, he remembered saying marriage needn't ruin a good friendship. Floy had been his best friend from the day they met.

Shirley was asking him a question: "So you have a son and a daughter. One of each. That's so nice. Did they play together when they were little, or are they too far apart in age?"

For the hard years, the hot summer years, the dust storm years, the impoverished years, there were just the two children. They transformed those years into the joyful years, the laughter years, the honeymoon years. Greg both liked and disliked his clerk's job at the jewelry store. He liked the customers, who recognized his love for and knowledge about the merchandise. He disliked the owner, who watched him hour by hour, as if waiting to catch his employee red-handed, stuffing precious jewels into his pockets.

For eight hours a day and a steady paycheck, Greg could ignore that. Once free for the evening or better yet, the weekend, he could hug and cuddle and tickle his wife and his babies. He could listen to their day's exploits—Larry actually sharing his sandbox dump truck with his baby sister, Judie adding to her vocabulary. "Bungy" was the newest word, deciphered when she pointed to a fly, a cricket, a wasp. To verify that bungies really were just bugs, and not all flying creatures, Greg pointed to a bird and asked, "Bungy?" His baby daughter shook her head decisively, saying "Bud," with the vowel sound like a German umlaut, or maybe the way a Boston Brahmin would pronounce "bird."

Life was good. Good things sometimes end, or change direction. The jeweler's customers were too few; sales were even fewer. In the midst of a nationwide economic depression, people do not have money for expensive trinkets. Greg was out of a job.

He studied the want ads, but there were few jobs that he seriously considered. Selling insurance in a poor economy is risky. He would not become a janitor. The government had just started programs intended to relieve the unemployment problem, the by-product of the stock market crash and the dust bowl years. And they were looking for educated men to oversee the programs. It would mean spending weeks at a time away from his family, but the pay was good, and Greg and Floy didn't have other choices.

He did not anticipate spending two years traveling the back roads of Idaho. His job was to visit government labor camps, verifying that the work was progressing on schedule, that the supplies were coming through on time, and that the camps were operated according to detailed specifications. There were several camps in Idaho, set up to house the workers who were building roads to connect isolated communities and provide access to wilderness areas. He vividly remembered the trek to one of them.

Just as he rounded a curve, he saw what had been a track wide enough for his car was now only half a track. That half was a narrow rut hugging the side of the mountain. The other half was a plank, spanning a gap of eight or ten feet over nothing. A mile below was the town from which he'd come.

Winding up the side of the mountain, mesmerized by switchback after switchback, he'd cursed the Civilian Conservation Corps. Not for the first time. But to be fair, the CCC was established to protect and improve the nation's parks and forests. The workers restored historical sites, built lookout towers and dams, strung telephone lines, planted trees, and set up tourist campgrounds and picnic areas. And they built the roads to make those places accessible. The road he was on was one of many such roads, barely worth the name, leading to hidden clearings in the nearly impenetrable high forests. The camp toward which he labored was in one of those clearings.

He debated momentarily whether or not to keep his eyes open while crossing over that puny half bridge—he couldn't turn around and go back, since there was no room to turn, and he could not back up through all those switchbacks. Then, slowly, he accelerated, eyes open, but devoutly praying. If he could do it going in, he prayed he could also do it coming out.

When he wasn't white-knuckling the steering wheel, Greg could immerse his senses in this country. So much water just burbling here and there and pooling in deep, dark, pure lakes. The lush green ground cover contrasted sharply with the land he had left—the parched farmland of North Dakota and Minnesota, topsoil blown away in the searing winds of those years that were sucking dry the souls of a million farmers.

The forests here could trade places with those of northern Minnesota and no one would notice. They were identical: mile upon mile of dark green boughs, raising their limbs in supplication to the skies for nourishing rain. The difference was that here, the forests climbed up and down, to and away from the timberline below the peaks of the surrounding mountains. Minnesota forests roamed up and down gentle hills. Both were balm to a solitary hiker; only the Minnesota ones were kind to a solitary car.

If he had expected a kindly welcome when he finally got to the camp, he had expected too much. He was met by a Kentucky mountain man, complete with shotgun cradled in his arms. Greg was not really surprised: the nation's unemployment was 25%, and the majority of those jobless men lived on the east coast and the southeastern hill country, not in Idaho. Only a quarter of the 115,000 CCC men working in the 51 camps in Idaho had homes in the state. So there were many men in Idaho whose families for generations had eked out a living in the mountains of Kentucky, wary of all who could not trace their ancestry back to those same mountains for at least a hundred years Greg hoped the mountains reminded them of home.

Someone else went to get the camp overseer while Greg and the mountain man silently waited, one not moving, with his eyes steadily focused on that shotgun, the other casually alert, finger on the trigger. After a few minutes—or an eternity—the overseer appeared. He muttered a few words to dismiss the mountain man and then observed. "Did you notice that that shotgun was aimed at your chest the whole time you were standing here waiting?" Yes, Greg had noticed. He was never sure whether there might have been a still on the property or if the guy was simply acting as he would have acted toward any stranger who suddenly appeared in his forested world. He didn't ask.

Shirley had asked a question: "You worked for Josten's, didn't you? My high school class ring is a Josten's ring. I still wear it, because it is so beautiful." And she showed him the lovely thing, a blue spinel in the center, with the school's crest in gold centered in the stone.

1937
Back home in a tiny, grubby town in North Dakota, Floy wrote chatty letters every week, including details about the children, the neighbors, the books she was reading, and the possible job prospects she had seen in the Fargo and Minneapolis papers, fortunately available in the town's small library. Usually, there were very few, and those few not very promising.

Finally, there was one that looked worth pursuing: a national company with offices in southern Minnesota, looking for a sales representative in North Dakota. The com-

pany manufactured high school class rings and a few other related items. Greg applied. He went for an interview with the president, Daniel C. Gainey. He got the job. He could go home!

In fact, Greg was euphoric, not just about the job and the opportunity to spend every weekend at home, but now they could move into a nicer home than the ramshackle place Floy and the children had endured and into a larger, nicer home in a larger, nicer town. They moved to Jamestown. The rent was reasonable, the grade school was close by, and life was, again, good.

"Your younger daughter will be here this afternoon—Jeannie is her name." Why did they keep telling him the names of his wife and children; did they think he was stupid? Did they think he had lost his mind? Had he lost his mind? His daughters still played cribbage with him, and he usually won because he could count faster than they could, so his mind must be all right.

1943

Jeannie. The blond, blue-eyed imp child who arrived when they could afford a child. Who arrived after they stopped reading baby-raising books that required new mothers to feed their babies no oftener than every four hours and not to pick them up if they cried before the four hours was up.

1966

Jeannie, whose wedding to Chris was such a happy occasion. Jeannie, who spent all summer every summer for many years looking after him and Floy at the lake, fleeing abuse that he had never suspected.

Jeannie's visits to him here—this hotel—were always the soothing same. She drove to the river—he wanted to stop by his mother's house. But he wasn't sure his mother had ever lived in Fargo. Jeannie stopped at the Dairy Maid ice cream store for sugar cones mounded with the world's best vanilla ice cream. Once in a while, Jeannie brought her dog.

1984

They were at the lake. Floy and Jeannie tried not to laugh, but that just made it worse. Jeannie finally left the room, barely stifling her giggles. Greg had always tried to remember to put his dentures in a safe place, one that he would remember. But some-

times the plate bothered him so much that it had to come out immediately, and he would just set it down in a handy place. And forget about it.

Dogs have a habit of noticing whenever anything that might be interesting is put within reach. Jeannie had Daisy with her. Daisy was sold by the pet shop as a beagle pup. Her coloring was beagle-ish, but when she grew up, her lineage was clearly Jack Russell terrier.

A dog of any breed might pick up an interesting-looking, accessible object. A Jack Russell terrier is guaranteed to do so. If a Jack Russell can create a scene, it will. Daisy had seen Greg put the offending dentures on an end table. When no one was looking, she picked them up. What set Jeannie and Floy off was the sight of Daisy prancing toward them, wearing Greg's teeth.

Greg did not find it funny, just further proof that women have a peculiar sense of humor. Greg loved Floy's rare but infectious peals of laughter. He only wished the target had been someone else. To be fair, that might have tickled his funny bone, too. For days after Daisy had pranced with his teeth, Floy had unsuccessfully stifled her chortles every time she looked at him.

Someone had come to visit an old lady he'd seen around the place, bringing a dog. Maybe it was the old lady's dog: she seemed really happy to see it, and the dog was wagging its tail and licking her face.

"I don't have a dog anymore," he said to the woman passing around a tray of cold drinks.

"Did you used to have a dog?" she asked, seeming interested.

"One of the kids did—nice dog, rust-colored."

"Would you like some iced tea?"

"I don't have a dog anymore," he told her, "but one of my kids did. It stole my teeth."

"The rust-colored dog?"

"What rusty dog? No. A little one with splotches."

"Was that your dog?"

"I don't have a dog anymore."

5

Perky Voices

Greg sometimes got tired of the overly perky voices of the nurses trying to get his attention, telling him to look at a visiting dog or someone's grand-kids. One of them was chirping at him, "Wasn't it lovely to have your grandchildren visiting with their little ones?"

"What grandchildren?" He was annoyed. These people kept trying to confuse him, to make him think his memory was faulty, to make him won-der if he was losing his mind.

The next morning, he woke up with a clear mind. He remembered the day and the visit and the children. He told Mrs. Hal all about it.

He'd been sitting in one of the lounges, just musing about not much of anything, when they came—Cathy and Wendy and their children. David was now a big boy of eight, a bit like Larry at that age, but more polite than Larry had been. He gave good hugs. Katie, his sister, was three and a half, a wiggly blond cuddler. She reminded him of his daughter Jeannie. Chelsea, Cathy's two-year-old, with her big, dark, danc-ing eyes, was like his memories of his older daughter as a toddler.

The little ones climbed into his lap, but like most small children, couldn't sit still for long. He thought they'd enjoy a walk after sitting in a car all the day before, so they set off for a trip around the neighborhood. He'd not noticed before how pretty it was with all the flowers in bloom. David held his hand while the two little girls, also hand-in-hand, picked dandelions. Their mothers vetoed assaults on the roses in one yard.

All grown up, Cathy and Wendy were still the dear granddaughters he'd known since they were babies. They were on their way to spend a week at the lake. He wished he could go with them.

A few days later, when Mrs. Hal was chatting with him about his family, she looked at the people just coming in the main door and said, "Your

granddaughters are here again with their children. How nice that they could stop in again."

Greg wasn't quite sure he knew who these two women were; they looked familiar, but his mind kept imposing images of children on these adult faces. The little girls weren't his daughters, although they looked a bit like some pictures he had. He caught a phrase "great granddaughters." It didn't matter. They were cute and quite willing to climb into his lap for a cuddle.

It was the boy he knew. Surely it was Larry, a bit shy as kids that age were—about third grade, he thought. One of those pushy women tried to join them. She was one of those people here who always seemed to want to horn in on everyone else's visitors (didn't she have anyone of her own?—not his problem.) He told her, not unkindly, but definitely, to go away and leave them alone. She was the bird's-nest-haired harridan who didn't believe he had had children visiting. He had told her they would be back. She finally gave up and went away when he told her, "See, I told you the boy would come back!"

He and the boy (one of the women called him David, which confused Greg; maybe this wasn't Larry, but a younger reincarnation?) talked a bit about basketball and the Minnesota Lakers, and the shyness disappeared. When they all had to leave and the boy said, "G'bye, Grandpa Greg," he understood for a minute that this wasn't his son. But that was okay—the boy was related to his son, and he looked like his son, and he was tall like his son, and the visit had been special.

He remembered another special visit from one of those children years ago.

1957
He had gone to the Winnipeg airport to meet Judie and seven-month-old Cathy after their 5000 mile trip from Yorkshire. Despite forty hours of riding in a car, a train, a transatlantic plane, and the plane from Montreal, Cathy was the picture of blooming health and delight, the happiest baby he had ever seen.

She greeted every new experience with crinkled eyes and baby gurgly smiles. Whether her internal clock stayed on British time or she just liked waking up with the sun, he couldn't tell, but every morning for six weeks she woke up at 4:30 and started talking to herself—or maybe to the squirrels pattering across the roof. After the first morning, when the dutiful mother had gotten up at the first peep and stayed up, thinking the baby might disturb the rest of the household, Judie got up, changed the baby's soggy diaper, and put Cathy in her pram on the porch, firmly shutting the door behind herself and going back to bed. Cathy continued gurgling and cooing at the birds and squirrels until the rest of the household were ready to face the day.

A few times, Greg got up earlier than the others and carried Cathy down to the lakeshore to watch the loons. She loved that. She loved everything.

She loved the taste and feel of Floy's oatmeal and baby-jar food. Floy had looked askance when Judie gave Cathy a baby-sized spoon and let her steer the oatmeal or peas or lamb or banana toward her mouth. Some of it arrived; more was smeared on her face and in her hair. Greg made an excuse to leave the room—if Floy saw him grinning at the joyous mess, she would be annoyed.

Greg suggested giving Cathy her baths in the old metal tub Larry and Judie had occasionally used when they were little, and putting it in front of the fire, which would be warmer than the tub in the bathroom. That worked for one bath; mops and rags dried off most of the floor, soaked by the exuberant splashes of a bath-loving baby. After that, the tub went out on the lawn at noon, to be filled from teakettles of hot water and cold water from the hose. Cathy got clean and the lawn got watered.

Cathy napped when it was nap time and didn't fuss when she was tucked in for the night—unless there was company. She loved a party. The Burgesses came over one evening to play bridge and, for the first time, Greg heard his enchanting granddaughter at her least enchanting—she howled. After a couple futile attempts to settle her for the night, they gave up. She was her usual sunny self as long as someone—preferably her doting grandpa—would hold her on a lap. Greg discovered it was possible to hold both a baby and a handful of cards.

Greg tried to tell his favorite nurse about the christening party, but he was finding it hard to think the words and harder still to make his mouth produce them. He could picture things in his mind, but the right words kept slipping away. He'd have to try to remember to ask Judie to bring the pictures he had taken that enchanted summer.

Judie had waited to have Cathy christened until he and Floy could be involved. Greg contacted the museum director to arrange the use of the museum chapel and one of its visiting clergy.

It was a lovely party. All the lake friends were there—Velma and Charlie Green, Beth and Ray MacKenzie, Gwen and Bill Franke, and a host of others. After the service—and a lucky photo of Cathy's wide-eyed look at the priest after he wet her head—there was a picnic lunch at the cottage. Cathy was due for a nap, and the rest of them could just sit and talk. But the guest of honor was not about to sleep though her party. After a couple of outraged protests from her crib, she joined the party and gleefully tolerated being passed from one lap to another. No nap that afternoon. She was a bit late joining the squirrels the next morning.

Greg recalled being too busy with the demands of his job, his investment properties, and their adults-only social life to spend more than two or three stolen hours at random intervals with his own babies or with his other grandchildren. Those few weeks with Cathy were memories he drew out of his mind often these days, just to relive and cherish, memories in which he was not just a bystander.

◆   ◆   ◆

Sometimes, Greg felt invisible. Floy seemed to avoid looking at him, and if there was anyone else with them, she talked to the other person, not to him. Riding one day with Floy and Larry, he realized they were talking—talking about, but not to him, as if he weren't there. He interrupted their chat, a bit amused, a bit annoyed, "I'm right here, you know, and I'm not deaf!"

Sometimes, though, he didn't hear the words people were saying, just a distant mumble. And sometimes he couldn't seem to make his mouth deliver what he was thinking. If he started to walk toward a door, people seemed to understand that he wanted to go for a walk, without the embarrassment of their saying, "I'm sorry, I don't understand" and his inability to express his wishes.

He liked going for walks. He remembered the long walks in the fields and woods near a house someplace he and Floy had stayed at one time—a long time; years maybe? When the kids came to visit, they'd go with him, loping across open areas—once finding the desiccated carcass of a cow. There were coyotes and maybe bears in that part of California, but he'd never seen one, just heard the nightly coyote choir practice.

He remembered slow strolls along the beach at the lake, from the cottage into town and back, stopping to visit with the familiar faces of long-time friends who were sunbathing or also strolling. Over time, it seemed, there had been fewer and fewer familiar faces.

Here, he took walks only if someone would go with him. The girls were good about that, seeming to understand that crossing a street had become a

fearful thing. They always waited patiently with him until no car could be seen in any direction. Greg couldn't remember when he had stopped driving, or why.

Floy rarely drove, even after she had her own car. She was a careful driver, but she found no joy in it, and she would not admit that she really needed driving lessons. Little bitty thing that she was, she invariably pushed the driver's seat back as far as it would go, so at 5'2", only her big toe had any hope of touching the accelerator or brake pedal. And she had to sit up, back ruler-straight (as she'd learned years ago in school, she had told him, from a teacher who actually did run a ruler up the spine of a slouching pupil), in order to see past the dashboard through the windshield. He did remember teaching each of the kids to drive.

Larry started taking the wheel at the age of twelve, when they went out to the farm for the Saturday horseback rides. Greg remembered surreptitiously borrowing a bed pillow so his son could see over the dashboard. It was only many years later that he heard about the Mounties chasing his son, with his endless supply of firecrackers, from the post office to the golf course, and later yet about Larry's verification that the new blue Oldsmobile ("the Blue Bomber") would indeed go 120 miles per hour.

Judie was a rules-of-the-road person, so he felt a bit guilty that he had not told her what power steering and power brakes did to the operation of a car. Fortunately, the car was parked heading out of the driveway, so all she had to do was drive out, turn left, and head for the farm. She drove out, turned the steering wheel to go left, and did a fast U-turn into the neighbors' driveway, just missing the tree growing on the berm. She slammed on the brakes, nearly putting them both through the windshield. Cars then did not have seatbelts. They sat there for a minute. Heartbeats back to normal, he asked if she wanted him to back out or would prefer to do it herself. It wasn't quite how he had intended her to learn the pros and cons of power steering.

Jeannie's turn. He would drive out to the farm, get his horse ready for a ride, mount, and lope off, telling his younger daughter to practice driving and turning and parking and accelerating and braking until he got back in a couple hours. She never hit anything, although he'd parked the car next to the barn. Before long, he let her drive back to town.

Jeannie was 16, with a brand-new driver's license, when he hired her to help Miss Wood, the manager of his resort and rental cottages at the lake. One of Jeannie's jobs was to pick up Mary, Sally, and other housekeepers who lived off semi-accessible, rutted back roads just outside the park, take them to the cottages ready to be cleaned and spiffed up for the next holiday renters, and then take them home again. After that summer, Greg figured Jeannie could drive safely and carefully anywhere.

Lately he had preferred having her or someone else do the driving, but he remembered how much he had enjoyed being at the wheel. Some people might find it odd that a person who drove a couple thousand miles a week for nine months of the year for his job still loved to drive.

1951

He had loved the summer when he spent six weeks driving his family on a tour of the western United States. It was a final gift of family togetherness. There was never another summer of all of them at the lake; there were no other travel tours as a family.

He remembered the pleasant conclusions of each day's drive. After marveling and taking pictures of Mt. Rushmore or the Garden of the Gods or Bryce Canyon or the Golden Gate Bridge, he had delighted in finding a really nice motel with, if they were lucky, a swimming pool so he could pack the kids off to amuse themselves while he and Floy found an ice supply, opened their portable ice chest for the bourbon and the beer, and had a loving, quiet hour to themselves.

Greg had a sudden clear image of Floy pouring over the AAA book, their travel bible, reading the descriptions of restaurants (what fun it was picking a winner, playing host to his family, and flirting a bit with the waitress) and comparing the options for overnight motels.

He remembered the morning routine: he and Floy would find a café for the essential cup of coffee, and a bakery and grocery so they could take sweet rolls and orange juice to the kids—Jeannie seemed to get less appreciative of sweet rolls and orange juice as the days went by. They also got fresh rolls and lunch meat either in that town or one further along the road for a picnic lunch, in a park, if they could find one. If not, they ate in the car as the miles disappeared behind them.

Freeways and rest areas didn't exist yet, so getting to places like Mt. Rushmore was a half day's drive around one hairpin turn after another, with glimpses, closer and closer every other turn, of those massive faces, tiny at first, barely showing through the evergreen forest, and always closer and bigger. He made Larry wake up and Jeannie get her nose out of her comic book to share the wonder. Floy and Judie were as captivated as he was.

Something had happened to his ability to know where he was going and how to get there. Maybe those few times he had gotten confused, he wasn't really lost; maybe he just hadn't gone far enough.

He remembered that they had headed out of Colorado Springs to see the Garden of the Gods, "just a few miles up that road there," they were told. The few miles stretched into ten and then twenty, into barren territory, not a house to be seen. The kids were getting fidgety, Floy was frowning, and he was getting concerned. Were they lost? And then there it was, that magnificent array of huge, red, stone formations, sculptured into incredible formations by the hand of God.

Greg would have been content to view only those place untouched by human hands, but he knew the kids needed a change now and then, so he took them to Los Angeles and a four-star Hungarian restaurant in the heart of Hollywood. They didn't quite drop their jaws, but their wide-eyed glee even before they looked at their menus was gratifying. He didn't admit that he had never eaten borscht before, either.

By now, restaurant dinners, unless really extraordinary ones like the Hollywood one, were beginning to pall. For a few days, they would cook their own. They'd previously arranged with Eddie and Harriet to rent a huge beach house on the Oregon coast.

Eddie was the only big brother around when Greg was little, too much older—5 years—to be a playmate, but kids grow up and do something—or nothing—and Eddie did something. He became an accountant. And he married a teacher. Quite acceptable enough for Floy, and it helped that Eddie looked like an accountant, not a farmer, He was thin, wore spectacles, had a neat, well-trimmed mustache, and looked a bit like Greg with a hint of Groucho Marx. Floy liked watching Groucho on TV.

Greg didn't think Floy ever knew Eddie's real name, which was just as well, since it would have been further proof that his family was weird. Who would ever burden a child with a name like Eugedean?

The adults were having fun playing cards and talking about people they'd known, interesting places they'd been, what it was like raising teenagers, and plans for the future for themselves and their children (Larry and his cousin Brice would be starting college in the fall, Larry at an elite, private, pricey small college at the other end of the prestige scale from Valley City Teachers' College and even NDAC. Greg knew his mother would have been proud.)

They were so engrossed that they didn't remember to call the kids in from the beach until it was too late. They did wish, not for the first time, that teenagers would occasionally show some of the common sense they were born with. All three kids got painful sunburns hunkered next to a pile of driftwood, freezing in the icy Pacific air but determined to get tan.

They all forgot that sun can burn even on a snowy mountain top; ask any skier. If she hadn't so very much wanted to be a part of the older kids' comradeship, poor eight-

year-old Jeannie would probably have left them and spared herself the agony of spending the next two days squirming in the car, unsuccessfully trying to make the sunburned backs of her legs comfortable.

Some western states were deliberately omitted from the tour. Greg knew that most of South Dakota, Nebraska, Kansas, Oklahoma, and Texas looked much the same as the great expanse of the mid section of North Dakota: flat, with torrid and tornadoey summers, frigid and blizzardy winters, and mile after boring mile of farm fields. It could be starkly beautiful in small doses; three days of driving to get to it all would be an overdose.

1955

Larry's wedding was in Texas, way south in Texas, in August before cars had air conditioning. It took nearly three days to drive from Fargo to Edinburg, through South Dakota, Nebraska, Kansas, Oklahoma and most of Texas. Floy sat beside him in the front seat. Judie, Jeannie, and a boy whose name he did not remember, a high school friend of Larry's who was to be one of the ushers, were in the back seat. They all sweated.

While they yawned through the boring, hot, dusty countryside, they all envied Larry, who was probably lounging in air-conditioned comfort or immersed in a swimming pool. He had flown to Texas a couple days before, since the wedding planner insisted that the groom needed to be available for a few days before the wedding. Greg wondered if her real job was to make sure the groom would be at the church on the right day.

At nine o'clock in the morning of the second day, they passed through a minuscule town in Kansas—one church, a bank, two bars, a general store, and a grain elevator keeping the few houses company. The thermometer on the local bank showed 109° and they counted nine funnel clouds thinking about touching down sometime that day. Greg couldn't remember what they ate on that trip, although they all remembered the air-conditioned restaurant at the hotel in Chickashaw, Oklahoma—and the non-air-conditioned rooms. Floy hadn't read the AAA book carefully enough. At 4:00 a.m. they admitted defeat—no one could sleep and they just wanted to get where they were going.

The accommodations in Edinburg were nice. The church, in Pharr, was nice. The bride's home in McAllen was nice. The country club in Mission, where the reception was held, was nice. The home of one of the bridesmaids in San Juan was nice. It was all very nice. Those places were all air-conditioned, and all but the church had pools. Each town was five miles from one or more of the others, so for five days, they alter-

nated between comfort indoors or in pools and discomfort in the car, driving to the next comfortable place. The marriage ended in divorce.

Larry's divorce so upset Floy that the Fargo house was sold and plans were accelerated for building the house in the hills around Julian. Greg remembered a wedding in that new house—Larry's daughter Lisa and a nice young North Dakota farm boy. Barb and Larry, as well as Judie, were there for the occasion.

Greg liked Barb. He'd also liked Susie, his son's first wife, Lisa's mother. He didn't like the groom's mother, who had accompanied the bridal couple on their drive to California and also accompanied them on the drive back home. Floy loathed her; she had absolutely no class. Bride-to-be, groom-to-be, and mother-in-law-to-be all traveling in the same cramped truck was one thing, but the witless woman also shared motel rooms with the couple both ways. That marriage also ended in divorce.

Floy and Greg were actually relieved about Judie's divorce. Greg never had liked or trusted that man—drank too much, dishonest, a freeloader. Jeannie's husband had liked him—maybe that should have warned them. They pretended for years that it was Jeannie's desire to look after them that kept her with them in Manitoba every summer; that Chris' job prevented him from spending even a weekend with them.

Reflecting on all that, Greg realized that none of their friends had ever been divorced. It just was not an option for their generation. He thought he had heard of one couple who divorced, but they left town separately and no one ever heard from either of them again. Even when a couple no longer even liked each other, they stayed together for the children, for the good of society. But they no longer shared a bed.

Thinking about that, Greg realized that Floy hadn't shared his bed for quite a while.

There was a time when she started the night in bed with him but, complaining of his snoring, moved in the wee hours into what had been the girls' room before they left home. And even then, they always shared a bed at the lake, until somehow he wound up sleeping in what had been Mrs. B's bed and then Jeannie's bed, and Jeannie moved into the other bedroom, leaving Floy alone in the lake bedroom—the one whose windows let in the gentle lapping of the waves as they came ashore, the one that they were to share forever.

That last summer, she had still said she loved him, but she seemed to shrink away from him, to choose activities that did not include him, to avoid the weekly gatherings of friends they had enjoyed for so many years. He had asked her what was wrong, but she never really answered. And he could not think of anything he had done to displease her.

And now he lived here and she lived someplace else and she visited him as if she were no more than a friendly neighbor.

September 1989– September 1990 Nursing Home: Third Year

"Memory isn't linear…only flicky-brief flashes where you can track through a sequence of events without skipping ahead, without finding other memories dragged in by association."
—James Alan Garner

6

SHARE THIS WITH ME

Greg wondered what the plans were for this summer. Except for the Western tour and the wedding, which had eaten up parts of two summers, they always spent three full months at the lake. Greg wanted to ask if they were all going to the lake this year when summer came, but he was afraid of the answer. He remembered being there with just Larry's boy, who was barely out of his teens and with an agenda of his own that didn't often include his granddad. Greg remembered missing his family, getting confused. He wanted to get that sour taste out of his head.

1939

He remembered the first real vacation he and Floy had, the first summer at the lake. At first, they were too poor to go anywhere. The school administrator's job allowed time in the summer to do things, but not the money to do anything with. Then Larry was born, and, 18 months later, Judie. Greg had changed jobs before they had to go on welfare, but the new sales job with a fledgling company was not yet making him rich. And vacations with two children in diapers are not really vacations.

Larry was six and Judie not quite five when conversation with a friend led him and Floy to three weeks in Manitoba, in a rented cottage on Clear Lake, named accurately, if obviously. The pine-ringed lake was deep and clear, and sandy-bottomed. He had never imagined deeps so pure, so like a window into a world of darting minnows and trophy-size cruising pike, and rocks of every color, looking as if they'd just been polished. From the squish-through-your-toes sands of the shore, or from a quiet rowboat on the lake, the cottages were virtually invisible, timidly trying not to spoil the seeming wilderness.

Accustomed to cabin-ringed lakes in Minnesota, filled with grab-your-legs weeds that frequently fouled the motors of the polluting speedboats belonging to summer people who seemed never to admire the lake and the trees and the sunshiny skies, but were forever rushing from nowhere in particular to some other nothing place in their shiny, new, unpaid-for cars and noisy, fast, unpaid-for boats—accustomed to that but not admiring it, he had never imagined a lake that was so cherished. He wanted to own this. No, one did not own this, one could only belong to this.

Molly Harrison owned the cottage next door to their rental cabin. Molly had emigrated from England in her teens. When Greg and Floy met her, she was in her early 40s, with four gorgeous teen-age daughters, one married son older than the daughters, and no husband. He had died, not much lamented by Molly, since for years he'd been carrying on an affair with Dr. Clark's wife. The Clarks owned the cottage next door on the other side of hers.

Molly had never lost her impressively upper-class British accent, nor her ability to swear like a mule-skinner without offending the tightest-lipped prude. Not that Floy was a prude, but she didn't swear beyond a rare "Damn!" and once, having nearly cut off a finger, "Shit!" Her oath of choice was the opening line of "Barbara Ritchie"—"Shoot if you must..." Even the kids knew she wasn't thinking "Shoot," just saying it.

Molly heard Floy's oath one day and insisted on hearing the rest of the poem. She thought her daughters might settle for a ladylike "Shoot!" if the alternative was a mouth washed out with laundry soap. Molly was a firm believer in "do as I say, not as I do." (Greg's own cuss word, which had his kids believing for years was a Norwegian oath, was "Sacramouche!" Greg had invented it one day as a French-sounding disguise for "son-of-a-bitch." Molly loved that one, too.)

She was determined to raise her daughters to be ladies and virgins until their wedding nights to the rich husbands their beauty would certainly snare. Floy and Greg enjoyed the nightly mother-watch as the parade of boys brought Molly's daughters home only seconds before curfew.

Each of the four did marry at the right time, to good-looking, respectable, comfortably-employed, if not rich, men. The day after the last wedding, Molly put her cottage on the rental list, and moved herself with a few furnishings, to the park campground. She was finally going to have a social life.

Molly visited often for a five o'clock drink, an evening of bridge, a dinner in or out. Floy rarely visited the campground; she was embarrassed to admit she knew anyone who would choose to live there, but Greg dropped in from time to time to join Molly and her new circle of friends in a quick game of matchstick poker or bridge, or to have a shot of scotch. One did not refuse to drink with Molly Harrison.

She was a brief house guest in Fargo occasionally. She loved shopping in the States—the quality was higher, the prices lower. Floy and Greg were tickled at her advice on how to get through the customs and immigration people with more money than the $100 the Canadian government allowed its citizens to take out of the coun-

try: *put $100 bills between the pages of a ratty-looking, rubber-banded diary, and swear—loudly—at any government official who made the slightest attempt to open that diary. Impudence and British hauteur will conquer every time.*

It would be fun to spend an afternoon with Molly again.

It was Molly who persuaded them to look at the cottage for sale on the other side of hers. Greg and the new company were doing well, but the budget was still very tight. He agreed to go look, but he had no intention of buying a cottage.

It was a real log cabin, chinks filled in with dried moss. In the main room, the gray-painted floors were furnished with a huge red picnic table and benches—the sort usually seen in picnic grounds, not homes; not even summer homes. A swing hung from the rafters in front of what would have been an attractive fireplace if anyone had ever cleaned it. Cheap, thin, garish curtains hung disconsolately at the windows: black background with enormous, fake-looking red and pink flowers and kelly-green leaves. Cushions covered with same fabric plopped on the ratty rattan chairs near the window where, if one stood up, one could see the lake. Unmemorable except for the grime were the bedrooms and kitchen that completed the layout.

Greg didn't see what was; he saw what could be. For $1000-nearly six months salary—the cottage could be theirs. Sitting up half the night with Floy covering sheets of paper with numbers while he thought out loud, they planned. If they rented the Fargo house every summer and stayed here, if he could do his summer paperwork here, if they were really frugal for ten years, if...

For the children it would be swimming and being cowboys and Indians in romps through the woods. It would be safe and exciting and away from the temptations of boredom and absent friends who had their own lake cottages. It would be three months, every year, of—vacation!

Greg knew he had been day-dreaming again. His cute blond daughter was here again, with her "Do you remember?" questions. This time, it was "Dad, do you remember how excited we all were every year when we started down the last hill toward the park entrance?"

He remembered. He coasted down the long, forest-fringed road to the park gates, traded his $10 bill for the windshield sticker that quietly announced the car was an accepted summer resident, drove past the outdoor roller rink that was waiting for the evening's skating teens, past Scrase's market and Meldrum's drug store and post office, *parking briefly in front of the Hudson Bay Company store (irreverently dubbed long since as the Here Before Christ store.)*

The brief stop was part of the traditional annual arrival. They all had to look at the lush lawns skirting the Chalet Hotel and the pathways through the trees to the vast sandy beach and the Main Pier, its slips filled with all sorts of boats bobbing impatiently, wanting, like Greg's kids, to get out to the lake.

Then he drove on, slowly cruising the mile and a half to their cottage, Floy and the kids noting who had painted or re-varnished their place since last year—and who hadn't, but should have. That half-yellow, half-green summer place had squatted between those two nice log cabins for years. The owners had repainted it once, in the same garish colors.

Squirrels zipped across the road in front of the car, barely avoiding suicide-by-tire as they had always done. Coming closer and closer to their driveway, they all leaned forward: Judie, Larry, and Mrs B with their chins nearly on the front seat head rests in front of them; Floy, Jeannie (who had to ride in front because she was prone to car-sickness), and even Greg with their foreheads nearly touching the windshield. And then they were there, home for the summer.

A staff person had gone around the lounge, telling all the residents that they would have to stay indoors for a couple of hours, because the outside patios had just been sprayed for mosquitoes. He told Floy that he hadn't noticed mosquitoes here, certainly not the size and voracity of those at the lake.

Until they settled in each summer, they tended to forget about the mosquitoes. Manitoba mosquitoes were humongous, their needle-noses bigger and more painful than the needles used in clinics to draw blood. And Manitoba mosquitoes seemed to drink more blood than any clinic ever drew from a volunteer. For a while, until DDT was banned, fogging trucks cruised the entire length of Wasagaming Drive about once a week. Cottage inhabitants were advised ahead of time to keep themselves, their children, and their pets indoors from ten until midnight on those evenings.

Floy asked, "Greg, do you remember the year that my brother-in-law made up several trial batches of insect repellent for us to test at the lake?"

Alex was an entomologist, a professor at NDAC. He and Floy's sister Hope and their daughter Jane Ann had spent a few days at the lake the year before, and Alex thought he could come up with a repellent that would disgust the insects. He'd con-

cocted three different test samples, each more obnoxiously odiferous than the last, for Greg to take to the lake.

The stuff repelled mosquitoes all right, but it also repelled any human or pet that got within five feet of the person wearing it. It was a toss-up which was worse: donating pints of blood to the mosquitoes and suffering middle-of-the-night frantic scratching, or lathering on Alex's repellents and keeping a breathing space away from other people, while hoping that your own olfactory nerves would cease to operate.

The owners of some of the new, large, elegant, very expensive summer homes had expansive decks, often on both the lake side and the road side. Their friends the Willoughbys had decks. Once or twice a year, they lit citronella candles and invited their friends over for happy hour. Generally, the guests were back inside in less than thirty minutes. Decks filled with people are prime hunting grounds for mosquitoes.

Florence Willoughby looked like she belonged in a new, large, elegant, very expensive summer home. Her looks were what are often described as "patrician"—elegantly coifed silver hair, carefully tended complexion, corset-contained body (Greg knew, because the Willoughbys were great huggers), and manicured nails.

Floy was very fond of Florence, but confessed to Greg that she was getting tired of Florence's references to her "large cans of beer," while she waved her small Manhattan glass. Maybe that was why Floy started pouring her beer into a glass, and finally stopped drinking beer and switched to Windsor Canadian and 7-Up.

Morley Willoughby drank beer; apparently Florence thought that was okay for a man. Morley did not look like he belonged in a new, large, expensive, summer home, with a living room larger than most entire cottages, so large the grand piano was tucked unobtrusively into a corner. He looked ordinary. Medium height, medium build, not much more hair than Greg had, nondescript features, pushing 70, and looking it. Morley owned one of the largest lumber companies in Canada.

Floy and Jeannie had started reminiscing with Greg about the summers after they met the Willoughbys. Greg had never been particularly interested in politics, as long as it didn't stick its nose into his business, but he remembered conversations with his Canadian friends that inevitably led to a discussion of government meddling, and the question, "What can we do about it?

Founding the Wasagaming Cottage Owners' Association was what Morley, Bob Hawley, and Greg had done about it. Morley was the first president; Greg, the second one. Their purpose was to get the Canadian government to pay attention to the collective voice of those who owned summer homes in Canadian national parks on land leased from the government. Originally, the renewable leases were for 99 years.

Recently, cottage owners in parks all over Canada had been informed that the law had been changed (without consulting them) to 42 years. Then came a plan to denude the parks of all cottages and open them only to campers—i.e., people with tents.

The outcry to Ottawa from Riding Mountain was joined by vehement protests from Jasper and Banff and other larger, older, richer and better known parks. The campers-only plan was shelved. However, the cottage owners across Canada realized the threats would continue, but they had power; they just had to organize it and start flexing their political muscles.

Jeannie and Floy asked Greg if he had enjoyed all those meetings of the Cottage Owners' Association and the public appearances he and the others had made to get as many people as possible involved. He agreed that working for a common good with people he liked and respected had been enjoyable. But then he remembered one duty that still embarrassed him when he thought about it.

Most of the work of the COA was worthwhile and gratifying. The Beautiful Baby Contest was not. The year he was president of the COA, Greg was conned into judging that event at the annual park festival. He had not realized that this was the original no-win contest for any hapless judge.

A dozen or so babies were all dolled up in sunbonnets and lacy dresses or, in the case of one boy baby, a miniature white tuxedo with an electric blue cummerbund that kept sliding into his diapers. One of the babies cooed and smiled. Most of them sobbed, yowled, howled, screamed, and/or threw up.

The babies, Greg could have dealt with. He could even pick out a couple that were better-looking than the others. Hair helped. Partially bald himself, he fully understood that a face framed with hair, curly or not, is more attractive than a fuzzless dome of skin.

It was the mothers who put the fear of God in him. Two or three were simpering at him while tweaking the cheeks of their offspring. Most of them were just glaring at him, daring him to pick a baby other than theirs. Greg realized, much too late, that he should have reneged, claiming flu or a heart attack or a dying grandmother. Whichever child he chose, he was doomed.

One family would leave with the blue ribbon, smiling but not surprised, since they knew from the beginning that Kootchy Karly was the most beautiful baby ever. But the other mothers, their husbands, their other kids, their in-laws, their aunts, uncles, cousins, grandparents, neighbors, and business associates would hate him forever, would shun him, would point him out at the grocery store and whisper behind his back. And they would never again support the Cottage Owners' Association.

After Jeannie stopped laughing about the Beautiful Baby Contest, she brought up some other memories. "Dad, I know that when I was really little, the cottage didn't have indoor plumbing or electricity, and I vaguely remembered a smelly outhouse between the cottage and the road. That must have been what you and your friends meant by 'roughing it.'"

For vacations, it was okay to carry drinking water from the spring down by the dock, haul pails of wash water from the spigot near the road and heat it in the teakettle on the wood stove, have the kids bathe and shampoo in the lake, suffer the indignities (and smells) of the outhouse, and store food in an outdoor icebox. The iceman came three times a week, lugging in his huge tongs another block of ice for the icebox that sat just outside the back door, ice that would melt quickly in the summer heat.

7

Memory is Not Linear

Three children (one a toddler), a one-hole outhouse, no running water, a tiny kitchen, and no electricity were making their summers difficult. Greg and Floy started making plans for modernizing some aspects of their vacation home, plans accelerated by a midnight visitor.

The elegant blond woman Jo Ann had introduced as his daughter Jeannie was still sitting with him out in the sunny patio at the rear of the hotel. She was talking about the lake—and the summer of the bear. He gave her a hug—he remembered a little blond girl name Jeannie. And he remembered the bear.

1948

They were all asleep when Greg was startled awake by what sounded like something banging the icebox just outside the back door. Quietly, so he wouldn't wake Floy, he tiptoed through the living room and into Larry's bedroom, where he could see the icebox outside the bedroom window. Even more quietly, he turned to wake the others, insisted on absolute silence. Jeannie was too little to see over the windowsill, so he picked her up.

It was a bear. A very large, dark brown bear, lying on its stomach with its head and part of its shoulders wedged in the icebox, the door of which was lying on the ground. Greg remembered the dinner ham had been in there. The creature emerged from the icebox and sat up. When they saw it holding the opened can of peaches in its huge paws and drinking the contents, they had to stifle giggles. Finally it ambled away, the remains of the ham in one paw.

Greg regretted what he had to do, but bears that get too cozy with the food supplies and garbage containers of park visitors and summer residents pose a threat. The next morning he reported the night visit to the RCMP post. By afternoon, the placid beauty of their small corner of the park was marred by a huge, green, wooden bear trap.

Two Mounties spent the evening drinking coffee and entertaining the kids with fabulous tales of Mounties—who always got their man—or bear—before they went to spend the night in their car in the driveway, watching and waiting.

For three evenings the Mounties watched while Greg and his family stayed close to the cottage. Walking the beach at dusk was not wise with a bear in the area.

The fourth night it stormed. Thunder, lightning, a deluge of wind and rain. Floy and the children fell asleep quickly, sure that the bear would not come in such weather. Greg was uneasy. He felt the bear was crafty enough to challenge the trap when watchers were least expecting it.

About 2 a.m., Greg was just nodding off in his chair. The sound was not thunder, but enraged roaring, splintering wood, gunshots, agonized bellowing. Finally, only distant thunder as the storm moved off. Greg grieved at the death of a wild thing that should have stayed in the wild, and went to heat up coffee for the weary Mounties.

Jeannie was still hugging him, bringing him back to the now. "It was the bear scare that led to the first improvements in the cottage, wasn't it, Dad? Indoor plumbing and electric wiring for a proper stove and refrigerator were first, weren't they?"

He remembered thinking how close they might have come to tragedy if someone had had to visit the outhouse the night the bear came. Yes, it was then that he had known they'd have to have an indoor bathroom, the sooner the better. And it would be nice to have an electric refrigerator that could freeze ice cubes.

1948–49

Plumbing and electricity were the top priorities, but if they were going to modernize, Greg decided it was time to enlarge the cottage and remodel it. Part of the addition was a new kitchen; the old one was converted to a bedroom for Mrs. B. and Jeannie to share.

He always called her Mrs. B. She understood that only one cherished person in Greg's life would ever be called or referred to as "Mother." His generation did not call their elders by their first names, so she couldn't be "Blanche"; his generation was taught respect before they learned their ABCs. "Mrs. B." suited them both.

He not only respected his mother-in-law, he genuinely liked her. She was good company, a slender woman who tried to look plain and unassuming, whose no-nonsense long hair was firmly braided every morning and pinned up, out of the way. She was quiet. She was not meek. Her dark eyes could twinkle or snap or ponder. Floy vehemently denied any Indian blood in her ancestry; Mrs. B. never said yes or no, but especially in summer, with a bit of tan on her gentle-stern, wrinkled face, she didn't have to say a word.

Mrs. B. never bragged, but when Larry jokingly challenged her to a rifle match one day, she beat the socks off him—ten shots, ten bulls' eyes. Once, she told how her husband had occasionally brought an unexpected guest for dinner and always bragged, with the after-dinner cigars, that he bet his wife could outshoot the guest. The wise guests begged off. The unwise took the bet, lost, and never again came for dinner.

That seemingly gentle, sheltered lady also played a mean game of cards. She taught the kids Blackjack, but not poker, although she once took on Floy and Greg at five-card-stud and won, of course. Evenings at the lake were often spent playing Hearts or Rummy.

Mrs. B. did not believe in letting children win; games, she felt, were for learning as well as for fun. She rarely lost. When she was dealt the queen of spades, she studied her hand and plotted how to dump it on another player's unsuspecting ace of some other suit or how to win with it and capture all the hearts. When the children won fair and square, she was as pleased as they were—and showed it. Mrs. B. was the best addition to the cottage, although the additional space and windows large enough to see through while sitting down had exceeded his hopes.

There was a new bedroom for Larry. And a screened-in porch, where Floy could sit, safe from the infernal mosquitoes, do her crossword puzzles, and read her murder mysteries.

For the new construction, Greg hired Dave Carter, a genius for building, repairing, remodeling, redoing almost anything, although he had never worked with logs for a major renovation. Greg remembered Dave telling him after it was finished that he would never again take on a job of building with logs—each log had required a full day's work from a team of four men. But Dave also admitted that he wouldn't have missed the experience.

Greg could still clearly visualize Dave Carter. He was a rough hewn man, always with a cheerful face, black curly hair, twinkly eyes, and a physique that attested to his years of hard manual labor. Like many Canadians, he had not gone to college, but he was well-read, and very well educated in reading people and working with ideas.

Greg liked and respected Dave, and he remembered his surprise when he realized that his wife, who did not normally treat workmen as friends, felt the same way. Even more surprising, Floy made friends with Dave's wife, who did their laundry. Greg remembered Floy admitting that, when Dave and Maisie came to Fargo one year for a few days' visit, she had expected the familiar drab-looking washerwoman in saggy housedresses and sockless feet in well-worn loafers.

Maisie on holiday was a different woman—salon hairdo, good clothes that fit properly, manicured nails, and high heels. And Dave, in a suit and tie and clean fingernails, was incredibly handsome. Greg didn't usually notice how other men looked, as long as they looked like everyone else, but he was used to Dave in flannel shirt and jeans, and he approved the transformation.

Greg thought somewhere he had a list of the projects he wanted Dave to tackle this year: the woodhouse needed attention. Dave and he had built the woodshed—built it properly of small upright logs about the circumference of Dave's forearm with spaces between the logs to keep air circulating and the firewood dry. But that last summer, the woodshed was alive with threats. He'd go in to collect armfuls of logs, and he could sense things, barely seen or not seen, slithering, flying, oozing through those open spaces. He could not bear having critters—real or spirit—nesting, hiding, lying in wait in the fireplace wood supply.

He remembered asking Dave to get him a supply of wood slats from a barn that was being torn down, and spending hours every day nailing up the spaces to make the woodshed critter-tight. The moss all over the logs within a week was annoying—the logs didn't seem to want to burn.

He'd heard Floy complaining to Jeannie about the mess he was making and the ugliness of the formerly woodsy-elegant woodshed. And he heard Jeannie's reply, "Mom, he's busy, he's happy, he's not just sitting in his chair staring unseeingly at the walls. Try to understand—when he's alert, he is grieving the creeping loss of his memory even more than you are."

He remembered hoping that particular memory would get lost, but it hadn't yet. It hurt. Or was he confused again? Didn't he remember that Dave had retired and his son had taken over the business? He wished his mind would stay on track, would stop blurring the then and the now. Memories were wonderful, but it seemed he had started living in them and was losing touch with the real now.

1960
He'd been thinking about the cottage renovations. He remembered the new fireplace that Curly had created after the almost disastrous fire, when Larry and a couple

college friends went up to the cottage during spring break and had such a roaring fire in the fireplace that when they woke up in the middle of the night, the mantle and the three logs above it were burning. What was it with that boy and fires?

He also remembered that, before an electric refrigerator was possible, when their after-dark light sources were kerosene lanterns and flashlights for trips to the privy, they had had to chip ice off the big block from the icebox whenever they had friends in for a little cocktail party.

Sometimes there was a cocktail party at this place. Floy always went with him and seemed to have a good time. Once she asked him if he remembered the old Canadian law forbidding liquor sales in national parks. He remembered.

If Floy and he wanted to serve drinks to guests, several trips were necessary to the nearest Leekybow (Liquor Control Board sales office) in Dauphin, 40 miles north, or Minnedosa, 30 miles south. Liquor could be brought into the park, one case of beer or one bottle of wine or hard liquor per trip, for home consumption only. Greg began planning how to get the law changed.

1950s
Greg remembered looking at the Rainbow Cabins, a sorry collection of run-down cabins painted in colors no rainbow would claim—unnatural greens and yellows, blues, whites, and browns, all grimy and peeling. They seemed to cower in the copse of trees, hoping the branches would hide their shame. Once again, Greg saw not what was, but what could be.

Floy's reaction to the inside of one of the shabby cabins was, "Oh, Greg, this is awful!" He was fully aware of the shortcomings: the chairs were not just unfit to sit in, they were plug ugly; a mouse had made a snug nest next to the flameless pilot light on the stove; the fridge was warm and smelled of mold; and the beds showed evidence of more mice using the mattresses as nests and potty boxes.

"Honey, you can not expect people to live with this."

"No," Greg had replied, "I'm going to transform it. You'll see."

Mooswa opened its doors a year later, dozens of sturdy new doors on dozens of woodsy brown guest cottages, no longer a hodge-podge of pointless dots of random, awful colors, but an inviting family of holiday homes, nestled in the woods.

Inside the doors, new furniture in cottagy fabrics welcomed guests, as did spotless, sweet-smelling refrigerators and clean stoves that worked. New mattresses on all the beds were mouse-dropping and lump free.

And Greg won his polite challenge to the Canadian government's law banning liquor sales in national parks, successfully presenting his argument to the political bigwigs that the serving of alcohol along with an elegant dinner did not lead to public drunkenness and obscene behavior.

He knew, although the Canadian government never would, that his persuasive oratory was due to years of persuading high school kids and their parents that a class ring was a worthwhile investment as well as a beautiful piece of jewelry; to years of presenting ideas to his fellow sales representatives; and most of all, to his speech teacher, Miss Sweeney, who had taught him how to breathe so long ago at Valley City Teacher's College. She would have been pleased.

Greg was pleased with how everything had turned out, but especially with the one new building that housed the office, a recreation room for rainy days, and, until other entrepreneurs got busy, the only dining room in the park where guests could have a cocktail before dinner and wine with dinner.

Provincial potentates honored Greg at the opening of Mooswa at a ceremony complete with an RCMP mounted patrol in dress uniform (those eye-stopping red ones) and all his friends. And his family. The glow of pride on Floy's face was all he needed.

1960s
And then he did it again, this time buying a derelict farm just outside the park boundaries that offered nothing except gently rolling hills and great views. Mooswa had almost everything people on holiday could want, but it didn't have a golf course, and it didn't have a riding stable.

Greg remembered seeing a painting in a museum someplace: a rolling landscape framed by a dappled forest of birch and pine, farmland once but now overgrown with weeds. The painting even had a ramshackle building, windowless, paintlessly gray, too stubborn to fall down.

He felt that he was standing just outside the site of that painting, and he could see what the painting did not reveal—spurts of wild wheat and brown-eyed Susans woven together in a carpet of bindweed with purple, lavender, pale pink blossoms the size of domestic morning glories. This was no painting. Light breezes carrying the scents of pine and horses and hay do not blow in a painted place.

Looking around, he knew where he would build the guest ranch and how the dining room windows would overlook the undulating hills of the golf course. The riding stable was already there, over to the east and far enough away that noise and smells wouldn't sully the guest rooms, but close enough for walking to.

Business at the riding stable was bad. The buildings were run down, unkempt; the manager was a surly, lazy drunk; the owner collected the rent and never came near. Greg would change all that. Holiday people loved to sightsee on horseback; all they wanted was a clean, inviting stable with docile, well-groomed horses and friendly, helpful cowboys as guides. That is what he would give them.

Greg proudly showed Mrs. Hal his yellowed copy of the <u>Winnipeg Free Press</u> article, complete with a picture of him with the Manitoba Tourism and Recreation Deputy Minister: "[They] rode to their job in style on Thursday afternoon as they cut a red ribbon to officially open the Elk Horn Guest Ranch, just a short distance from Wasagaming in Riding Mountain National Park...[Greg], president of Wasagaming Properties Ltd., a North Dakotan who saw the potential in a guest ranch operation in the park, has build the [$N] lodge—with modern accommodations for 96 guests—and plans to operate it on a year-round basis, with skis and motor toboggans taking over in winter months from the horses..."

Greg was glad he had that clipping; he didn't remember the skis and toboggans (and wasn't there a golf course, too?) until he pulled the clipping out of his wallet again. He had forgotten the plaque with the engraving: "1969 The Rex Grose Award Presented annually for Outstanding Merit in the field of Tourist Accommodation and Visitor Relations in the Province of Manitoba."

8

HORSES AND HOLIDAYS

He was glad there were horses at the lake. He loved horses. He had been around horses most of his life, and he remembered each one. If he shut his eyes, he could see them.

1944

Lady was a nice, ordinary, bay quarter horse with a white blaze, white feet, and black mane and tail. Midnight, Larry's horse, was part Hambletonian, solid black, a well-mannered, unexciting mare. Judie's horse, Red—a bay gelding—had manners, but only with Judie riding him. He patiently stood while she used a mounting block to scale his 17-hand height. He was a very big horse for a little girl.

If anyone else tried to mount Red or ride him, Red forgot all the manners he ever had, fidgeting and dancing around until the would-be-rider was thoroughly exasperated. Even that behavior was tolerated, because he was so good with his 10-year old rider. But Greg finally got tired of being called out from town to the farm a mile down the road from his place, to lead Red back to his own barn. Red was a hunter-jumper, so he could soar over the gate of his tie stall, amble out the barn door after checking that no one was looking, and trot off to visit the neighbors.

Red had to go. His new owner wanted a hunter-jumper, and she got a jumping wonder. Red was not Greg's idea of a wonder horse, nor was Lady or Midnight. He had seen his ideal at sales school.

As salesman of the year, Greg had had the honor of presenting his boss, his friend Dan Gainey, with a true "drinker of the wind," a stallion imported from Arabia. That elegant, ruler-of-the-world head raised in challenge and curiosity to the winds of his new home. That sleek, powerful, graceful body, sheathed in a coat already turning to silver. Those surprisingly soft, near-black eyes, alert, not alarmed, their color repeated in the lush mane, forelock, and tail. And all ballerina-balanced on such seemingly delicate legs. This horse was poetry, legend, an unattainable dream.

"Was that your horse?" asked a visitor, pointing to a painting of the head of a soft-eyed, silver and black horse on Greg's wall.

When he had made that presentation to Dan, Greg had vowed that someday he would own a son of that incredible stallion. Three years later, he took Gai Dei home. There had been horses all his life—horses he'd raised and trained and ridden for himself and others. There had been mutual trust and respect. With Gai Dei, there was more: an almost telepathic bond.

Greg loved riding Gai Dei in parades and equine shows, demonstrating the oneness of horse and rider by laying the reins on his knees and guiding the horse through a pattern of poles with just his legs and his mind.

"Not <u>was</u>! That <u>is</u> my horse. He is an Arabian stallion." Greg flatly rejected the fleeting memory of a long-ago phone call requesting permission to put Gai Dei down. He had slipped and fallen on the ice of his winter pasture and smashed his thigh bones. Nothing could be done.

"Tell me about your horse, your Arabian stallion," his companion asked.

"Have you ever seen a weanling foal?"

"What's that—like a colt?"

Greg explained. "A male foal is a colt, a female foal is a filly; foals are baby horses. A weanling is a three-or four-month old foal that has just been weaned."

"I don't think I've ever seen one that young."

"You haven't. You'd remember if you had. Imagine a mini-sized horse's body balanced on unbelievably slender, graceful legs that seem to account for two-thirds of the animal's height—you measure a horse from the ground to its withers: the back, right below where the neck starts.

"Imagine the straws of a broom that has lost any shape it ever had as well as half its size—that's the foal's tail, almost constantly twitching, in fun, at flies, or just because.

"Then imagine the head of a mature horse, only smaller, but leave the ears adult size. Then imagine the eyes. A foal will flirt with its eyes; may roll them at you, showing the whites; may bat the eyelashes at you (the longest, lushest eyelashes God ever created.) After you have demonstrated that you pose no threat, it may direct a liquid gaze into your eyes. It's like looking into each other's souls.

"You can't imagine what a foal feels like without actually touching it. The nose area is like velvet, but warm, alive. The coat is like fine satin if you stroke it one direction, like suede rubbed the other way. After that, the coarseness of mane and tail come as a surprise. Neither looks like anything other than a bad haircut. The mane isn't long enough to lie nicely along the side of the animal's neck, as it will later, so it just sticks up, all spiky. Looking at a weanling foal, you want to laugh at the comic touches, and weep at the sheer beauty of everything else."

The man interrupted, "Mr. G, you were going to tell me about your Arabian stallion."

"I just did tell you about him, about what he was like the day he arrived at the farm. Gai Dei gingerly backed out of the trailer, pirouetted to look over his new home, and pranced up to me as if to say, 'Have we met?' I loved him from that moment on."

Greg had not owned horses of his own for many years, but he remembered being invited for rides with friends. He vowed he would never forget the invitation to spend a weekend in Arizona at the Gainey ranch, reminiscing, riding, and watching an Arabian horse auction.

One of the girls had brought the letter he had written about that unforgettable time:

"...Dan was standing across the ring. [He] turned and saw me and welcomed me with open arms. After a brief visit he took me to the guy with the mike, and introduced me, in glowing terms, as the man who had presented him with his first Arabian.

"The auctioneer, his two helpers, the grooms, the ring masters were all in formal dress. There was a band, about 2000 spectators. The lights turned out and a spotlight followed each horse as it was led in by the groom, then lights turned on and the Arabian was turned loose. Such beauty!

"Before the horses entered, after the auctioneer had stated the rules, Dan got into the ring and said, 'You came here to see champions. Before you see the horses, I want you all to meet another champion, my friend [Greg].' [Dan] again told about my presenting him with his first Arabian, and then had me stand and had the whole crowd stand. I was the only person that sat with the Gainey families. It was some experience. Signed autographs yet.

"It is kind of patting myself on the shoulder, but I thought you would like to share this with me. Love, Dad, Grampa." [dated February 7, 1975]

Floy hadn't been there to share the glory with him, but he thought he remembered telling her about it.

◆   ◆   ◆

Floy was trying to make conversation, to wake up his sleeping senses: "Greg, look at the beautiful Christmas tree and all the lovely decorations around the doors. Christmas is always such a special time."

1938

Greg had almost forgotten the Christmas when the two kids were little, when he'd started to be recognized as his company's top sales rep. A medium-sized, but extremely heavy box had just arrived from Mr. Gainey, the president of the company, addressed to Mr. and Mrs. G. and, in capital letters, AND CHILDREN.

He put the box on the bed and carefully cut the tape, and reached in to pull out the contents—small, surprisingly heavy bags that jingled. Larry and Judie watched, wide-eyed. He opened one and dumped the contents onto the bed. It was loaded with—pennies! Mint-shiny pennies! Floy and he were now as wide-eyed as the kids.

They started counting, and they all giggled when they lost count, more than once. Finally they developed a system—each of them would put 10 pennies in a separate pile. There were 10 piles—100 pennies. One dollar's worth of shiny new pennies. None of them had ever seen so many pennies.

The children were eager to start dumping out the contents of the other bags in the box, but Greg suggested that they put all these pennies back in their bag, check the contents of the other bags, and then just count bags. A bit disappointed, but seeing the sense in that approach, they all started stuffing the first bag. Then they started pulling out the others.

Greg's eyes got even wider as he began to realize just how many bags of pennies there were in that box. He had been so worried that Christmas that year was going to be a disappointment for the kids—one item of clothing for each, one book, and one cheap toy was going to strain the budget, and he and Floy had already decided a chicken was the best they could afford for Christmas dinner. There were oranges and apples for the Christmas stockings.

They were all grabbing bags of pennies from the box and putting them on the bed—Greg's eyes got wet as he saw that they were stacking the bags in groups of ten. There were ten piles of ten bags each. His struggling company with its confident owner, a man who was becoming a good friend, had given him and his family the best Christmas of their lives.

Greg hugged the old lady sitting beside him. She looked surprised, but pleased. She was saying something, and it was important, so he strained to understand. "Greg, they're serving hot cider in the lounge. Shall we go join them?" She looked a bit like Floy when they had people over for a Christmas party. This was Floy. There was something really wrong with his head. But he smiled at her and got up—and remembered.

The house was full of friends, neighbors, and kids—his and everyone else's. He was in the kitchen, attired in his chef's hat and apron—gifts from the kids last year, when they had decided that for this annual occasion, he needed to have the proper accoutrements.

This was the Tom and Jerry party, held every year on the Saturday before Christmas Eve. The secret recipe, all foamy and rich, was whipped ready in a huge bowl. The kettle was boiling. The Tom and Jerry mugs (a gift from someone a few years ago) were lined up on the counter, a shot of bourbon in each, waiting for the boiling water to be poured gently over, leaving lots of room for the foam on top—with a dash of nutmeg to complete the work of art.

Kids over 18 were allowed one mug, and only one mug. Little kids got a mug with cocoa instead of bourbon and water, topped, of course, with the secret recipe foam and the nutmeg.

And then the toasts—to Christmas and babies and promotions and peace and goodwill to all men and women and children. Everyone sipped—the drink was too hot for anything else, and there was no danger of anyone having too much to drive home after the festivities. Greg loved playing host—and his lovely wife (God, she was lovely! that dress, that shape within the dress, those sparkling eyes, that happy mouth!) was having a marvelous time, surrounded by those who loved her.

Sipping her hot cider, Floy chatted with strangers and exchanged holiday greetings. Floy was looking more like herself, he thought, smiling at people and comfortingly holding his arm. He just kept smiling; couldn't think of anything to say. She hadn't seemed that happy recently. The cider was okay, but it wasn't his favorite drink.

The Prohibition gin stirred up in the ATO bathtub wasn't anyone's favorite drink, but the thrill of keeping it hidden made it special. They didn't often have access to anything else, although once in a while someone made a run to the border and smuggled back a bit of real liquor. Prohibition was only a minor nuisance to young people who weren't much into drinking anyway. The gin, in lots of orange juice or cider, was okay for parties—in small amounts.

After they were married, Greg remembered, there was no money for liquor, even if anyone had wanted it. By the time Prohibition ended, there was still no money for such things. But by the time FDR's New Deal got going, and the dust bowl states were seeing some welcome rain, and the stock market was rallying, so jobs were more plentiful, he had the new job. The household budget was still carefully revised every weekend, and needs came first, but once a month someone in their group of friends hosted a party, and everyone brought whatever contribution they could afford.

Cheap bourbon mixed well with 7-Up and other mixers—and the morning after a party at their house, Greg and Floy loved watching Larry and Judie check out the kitchen to see if there was leftover "mimorkey." They loved the stuff. To them 7-Up was for sick tummies, so this was the only soft drink they knew, and they thought it was ambrosia. As he recalled, it was Judie who had come up with the name, unable to pronounce "lime rickey."

She sat down beside him, after giving him a big hug—he loved this daughter who looked so much like his wife. "Merry Christmas, Daddy! I brought you a present. It's a photo album with pictures from that Christmas when I was fourteen, when you and mom took me to Chicago. Let's look at them together." She opened the book to the first page and time skipped backwards.

1948

Judie's Christmas present had been his idea, Greg remembered. He had a sales meeting in Chicago; Floy and Judie could shop and visit museums during the day while he was busy, and they could all do something special in the evenings.

For Greg, trains were a rare, pleasant break from driving, and the Vista Dome from Minneapolis to Chicago was a special treat. Only the truly blasé would stay in the lower part of each coach, asleep or reading. Greg led his wife and daughter up the few stairs to the upper, observation level, where the roof of the coach was a glass arc, granting full views of the surrounding scenery.

As dusk fell, lights came on in every direction—not just ordinary street lights, but all the Christmas lights of the Twin Cities and all the little towns along the way. And the lights of the stars, which waited to sparkle in the dark areas between towns.

The train sped past fields and pastures and forests to the Wisconsin Dells. Barely visible were the magic rocky peaks and valleys with the river spearing and disappearing below. On through more fields and much busier highways, with different lights, the moving lights of cars as tiny as fireflies. Long before the train slowed, the glow in the sky from the lights of Chicago spread across the sky. And then they were there, bundling off the train, greeted by a small group of men who hugged him and Floy and graciously kissed Judie's hand. She almost curtsied, she was so thrilled.

Into a taxi, off through a kaleidoscope of lights, swooshing up to the door of the Palmer House. His daughter had never seen a doorman before. An elegant hotel, royally gussied up for the holidays, with a palatial suite for their stay. They just had time to change for a late dinner. Dinner at their house was always at 6:00, but high society, of which, for a few days, Greg and his family were a part, dined at 9:00.

Judie was promptly adopted by the waiter who had only her mother and her to take care of—Greg knew she had never seen elegantly dressed black men serving meals before—mostly just young farm girls earning a bit extra for marriage or—rarely—college. The man called her "Miss Judie," and she basked in the attention from him, and also from the friends of her dad's who made a point to come and chat. If only his mother could have seen this, Greg thought.

Back at the hotel each afternoon, Greg briefly recounted his day at conference sessions, and then listened with joy as his wife and daughter bubbled about shops and shop windows. His daughter painted him a word picture of a Marshall Fields' window, with life-size, moving manikins in red, blue, green, white and silver costumes, skating around an icy glass rink rimmed with evergreens.

And Carson, Pirie, Scott had a whole family of life-sized Teddy bears that moved around their Teddy bear house, mother bear cooking in the kitchen, two bear cubs having a pillow fight in a bedroom, daddy bear reading a newspaper in the living room.

Starry eyed, she told him about racing across the Outer Drive in Chicago's icy winds with her mother, both giggling like schoolchildren let out for recess, to get from the Planetarium ("Daddy, they showed us what the sky was like 2000 years ago, and what the Star of Bethlehem might have been!") to the Natural History Museum ("lots of dinosaur skeletons—you wouldn't believe how huge!")

Floy's coup of the day was tickets to "South Pacific." His wife was a marvel at talking box office denizens out of tickets that didn't exist. "South Pacific" had been sold out for months.

Greg remembered that he and Floy had never let on to his daughter that this was their first Broadway musical, too, and that their evening had been as enchanted as hers. For a few minutes, looking at pictures of long ago with his arm around his daughter, Greg's mind was clear. He was tired, but it was a nice kind of tired. Judie had to leave, so they hugged, and he slept.

◆   ◆   ◆

One set of Christmas memories overlapped and merged with others, so Greg wasn't sure which year it was that Mrs. B. overdid the brandy. It wasn't her fault. But it still made him smile.

"Mom! Dad! We have oranges in our stockings!" Christmas Day always started off the same, with the kids waking up the whole household as soon as they had checked out the contents of their hearth-hung stockings.

Greg figured that every family with parents who had endured relative poverty as children had told their children how tough things had been and how grateful they had been for the once a year treat of an orange. It had become the joke of a generation of families, right up there with walking five miles (or was it ten?) to school every day, in howling blizzards. The kids were surprised that dad never mentioned wolves.

Except for Larry, all were in bathrobes. Larry sneered at bathrobes and wasn't old enough for dressing gowns, so he had stuffed his Flash Gordon pajama tops into jeans.

Judie, with her new page boy hairdo, including the bangs she had been pestering about, looked less than elegant in last year's now frankly tacky, faded blue chenille bathrobe. Every Christmas enhanced her wardrobe with a new one; this year's would be a bright coral.

Jeannie was already demonstrating a keen fashion sense—her lavender terry robe had matching slippers and a headband over carefully brushed hair.

Floy wore that bright red robe he had given her last Christmas, the one she would wear faithfully once a year for many Christmases to come. Under it was an old, once lovely, now too-often-washed silk nightgown. Under their bed were boxes of never-worn nightgowns that Greg had bought for her, "too pretty to wear for everyday."

Greg suddenly remembered that the tornado years later had snatched all those boxes, and after that, his wife (who looked stunning in the lingerie he bought for her) started wearing his gifts on ordinary nights—which then were not so ordinary.

There was a new silk confection for her under the tree that year, too, but it wasn't her turn yet. Present opening took a lot of time. Greg didn't remember how it started, but he would pick up a brightly wrapped box, check who it was for, and hand it over to be opened. After everyone had admired that gift, the recipient picked up and delivered the next one. So one by one, the gifts were opened and admired; the pile of dis-

carded boxes, ribbons, and wrappings grew higher and higher; and so did the treasure hoard next to each person.

Then breakfast. No oatmeal on Christmas, but coffee, cocoa, and rosettes—those inch-high stars of wafer-thin pastry, deep-fried and then dipped in powdered sugar. They ate at the table in the utility room to avoid a shower of sugar powder all over the recently vacuumed dining room carpet and the freshly polished table.

Now they had to get to work. Gifts were nestled back under the tree, ready to show off to visitors. Bedraggled gift wrappings were unceremoniously stuffed into a large box and put out of sight for trash pickup.

Jeannie's job was tearing bread into pieces and chopping the celery and onions. She had been allowed to add the sage and poultry seasoning since she was old enough to use measuring spoons.

Greg gave the turkey a final rinse, inside and out, and paper-toweled it dry, while Floy greased the huge roasting pan. Larry peeled potatoes, muttering (with a grin), "Might as well join the army." Judie set the table with the special occasion lace tablecloth, the matching napkins (no paper on this special day), and the sterling silver tableware, carefully polished just the week before.

Greg held the bird while Floy stuffed its innards with the bread dressing, lifted it into the roaster, and hoisted it into the waiting oven.

Hors d'oeuvres were ready, potatoes and other vegetables were in their pans on the stove, pies were waiting in the fridge, the rolls just needed a warm-up. Time to get dressed and welcome the rest of the family.

If the kids had helped get dinner ready, why did he remember Larry arriving with Susie and their two or three or four children? And Judie coming with that man and Cathy and Snookie Poo? (Was Wendy too old for the pet name?) Jeannie didn't come at all—she was with her husband at the Minot Air Force base. Mrs. B was the only one who never seemed to age.

People might change, but for Greg, Christmas didn't. Every year it was a houseful of people laughing and hugging and talking. And one year, Greg had opened some brandy for after dinner with the coffee. He poured a snifter for his mother-in-law, reminding her that her doctor had said a little brandy or port after dinner would be good for her.

Some time later, they all realized that Grandma was not in the room. They looked all over. Floy found her, sound asleep in the guest bedroom. Greg teased Mrs. B about it—once. She gave him the look that mothers give to small boys who have overstepped the boundaries. It was never mentioned again.

September 1990– September 1991 Nursing Home: Fourth Year

"Dear God, I didn't think orange went with purple until I saw the sunset you made on Tuesday night. That was really cool."
—Thomas

9

WINDOWS

Greg woke up to the sounds of the approaching storm, and shuffled over to the window to watch. He'd always rather liked storms, unless he was right in the middle of them, and this one looked like a doozy. From a clear, unruffled blue, the sky had rapidly turned cloudy, then darker and darker shades of gray, and finally an eerie, vicious green. The wind had come out of nowhere, suddenly whipping the trees in frenzy, as if to rend them to splinters.

He had a front row seat and was annoyed when one of the white coats interrupted him and told him they had to go downstairs. There was nothing downstairs he wanted to see, just the activity room whose activities he had never found interesting. There were no windows down there, and he wanted to watch the storm. At least he did until someone shrieked "Tornado! We'll all be killed!" and began sobbing hysterically. Several white coats bundled the person away.

Now he was concerned. Where was Floy? They had to get to the basement!

1947

She was with him on a short drive, to mail a letter to Judie and to see if they could spot the tornado the radio announcer had said was sighted near West Fargo. They'd seen it, all right, dark, ugly, huge, powerful, maliciously threatening—and heading toward them, less than a mile away. They could see the debris of what had been trees and homes whirling in its maw. Greg wheeled to race for home and the shelter of the basement.

They shut the basement door, scurried like frightened mice down the stairs, and huddled near the furnace, holding each other tight and praying. They couldn't hear themselves; the noise above, around, through them was as if they were inside a freight train, out of control and careening to disaster. As suddenly as the din started, it stopped. The quiet was as frightening as the tumult.

They waited. The quiet continued. Claustrophobia was closing in. They inched up the stairs. The den looked untouched, as did the utility room. They opened the door to the kitchen, and saw the open sky over the dining room and through where the living room wall had been. The chimney was poking through the living room ceiling, through the floor of what had been the girls' bedroom. They went outside. The roof was gone, most of the second floor was gone, half the first floor was shambles.

One by one the neighbors emerged from their homes. The house on the corner had only a broken window. Only the basement remained of the houses next door on either side of theirs. At the very end of the block were two homes that looked whole. The only three houses across the street were destroyed. But the people were all safe, and gradually, one by one, they moved toward one another. They were neighbors.

People were running toward them from all directions to gawk, to help. And there came Larry, frantic eyes in a sheet-white face, looking for them. Greg had not realized until that moment how much his son loved him.

When they'd all caught their breath and dried their tears, Larry told them he had heard on the news that the tornado had ripped a path five miles long and eight houses wide between 13th and 14th avenues. Fearing the worst, he had driven the four miles of winding gravel roads from the farm in less than four minutes, only to be stopped by a roadblock on 14th Avenue. He had abandoned the car to run toward home, toward his parents, toward a grief he did not think he could bear.

After terror, after relief, after euphoria that only things had been lost, not lives, practicality surfaced. Insurance would repair walls and roof, would replace furnishings. But a quick inventory revealed the irreplaceable lost: Floy's rings. Their monetary value was negligible, and insurance would cover that. It could not return the rings.

When Greg proposed to Floy, he told her that some day, he would shower her with diamonds, but for now, he could only give her his heart. Her wedding ring was a plain band of white gold. For their fifth wedding anniversary, he gave her the belated engagement ring, the best he could afford, a quarter-caret stone in a simple setting.

Floy had been doing the dishes when they'd suddenly left to see the tornado encroaching on the city, leaving her rings on the what-not shelf near the sink. The tornado had stripped the shelves of the little Spode vase with pansies in it, two or three ashtrays filled with buttons and safety pins, a Royal Doulton cup and saucer from Molly Harrison, and the rings.

Realizing they were gone, Floy was in tears—his beloved wife who never cried. Greg felt like weeping himself. The rings were more than metal objects, they were memories and promises.

After Larry and a group of his friends had blanketed the naked top of the house with tarps, to keep out the rain that followed on the heels of the tornado, Larry borrowed a flashlight from someone and began slowly quartering the front lawn and the neighbors' lawn. Within minutes, the flashlight beam picked up the sparkling reflection from a diamond nestled in the grass. A closer look revealed both of Floy's rings. No safety pins ever turned up.

The old lady who said she was Floy was there again. He liked her, and sometimes he believed her. She was asking if he'd seen the tornado that had skipped over the city. And then he knew she was Floy, because she said, "Do you remember the drapes?" And for the first time in what seemed like a long time, they gently laughed together.

When they'd first bought the house and essential pieces of furniture, there wasn't much money left over for proper draperies, so they made do for a while with inexpensive curtains. But later, they could afford to redecorate. Half the fun was pouring over books of fabric samples together, trying to picture what that scrap of material would look like as living and dining room drapes. The final decision was the most beautiful pair of drapes they'd ever imagined, a cream background with a pattern of bamboo poles entwined with dark green, long, slender leaves and dark crimson petals the same shape as the leaves.

Once every year or two, Floy asked if he thought the drapes should be cleaned, but they both feared the fabric might be damaged, so they postponed it. The elegant drapes had been adorning the windows for at least ten years when the tornado hit. At first glance, they seemed to have survived, but they were filthy and embedded with tiny shards of glass.

Larry and his crew of friends carefully took down the drapes and bundled them off to a cleaning shop that specialized in fire, smoke, and water damage. When Floy and Greg heard the assessment, they had to laugh—the proprietor of the cleaning establishment informed anyone who would listen that the only thing holding those drapes together even before the storm was a decade of unseen dust. The cleaning solutions had left clean tattered shreds of crimson and green glory.

Shreds—where had that word come from? Plans in shreds? Brain in shreds? He wanted to ask, but he was afraid of the answer, and when he

thought he'd asked, "When can we leave for the lake?" her blank pitying look told him she had not heard those words nor any others she could make into sense.

1946

Now he remembered: they had not been able to go to the lake for a couple years, but finally the war was over, gas rationing was over, the baby was old enough to enjoy the lake, and they could go!

He took the two older kids up as soon as school was out. Before Floy got there with the baby, he wanted to get the dreadful gray-painted floors sanded, suspecting there was a beautiful hardwood floor under all that gunk. A week of work and play with the older kids would be a pleasure for them and for him, and his wife would enjoy a week of peace with just the baby to tend.

The ice in the lake was in its final breakup as they drove north. When they arrived, they dashed down to the shore, as they had always done, to make sure nothing had changed. Small icebergs piled willy nilly along the entire shoreline—it was like an alien landscape; it was magic.

Greg had heard about the other worldly aura of icebergs, chilling not just bodies, but the minds of those who came near. He knew ocean-faring bergs were enormous, the visible tops rivaling or surpassing multi-storied ocean liners, with most of their vast bulk lurking hidden under the ocean swells. One of these, by comparison, was tiny, and fully visible, beached like a careless whale.

Yet many were larger than the canoes and rowboats safely awaiting the return of their summer people, in their protected boathouses or under their owners' cottages. And these diminutive fortresses of ice, like their giant cousins, emanated, not malice, but menace.

His son and daughter, too young to sense the menace, were simply amazed that the forces of nature could make ice castles and tunnels and forts that were bigger, better, solider than kids could create in a whole day of shaping blizzard-made snowdrifts. Greg wondered again, as he had in the past, if kids really did not have nerve endings, did not feel the paralyzing cold.

The kids were at the lake, so of course, they had to go swimming the next day. And Greg felt honor-bound to go in with them. Trying to ignore the fact that the water temperature was probably no more than 35°, and knowing that if he put a tentative toe in first, he'd never get the rest of his body in, he trotted to the end of the dock and dove in. He couldn't breathe! But the kids had jumped in after him, and he couldn't let them all turn into ice statues, so he swam for shore, grabbed the pile of towels, and wrapped up his children before they all ran, teeth chattering, to the cottage. He had had the sense to get a good fire blazing before they left.

Floy had been very pleased with the floors. They'd waited until mid-June before going back, knowing the lake would be about as warm as it ever got and that all the park facilities would be open.

The baby, now a three-year-old, thought this was heaven. She was enchanted with the squirrels that dashed fearlessly up and down trees right in front of her. She loved paddling in the lake and building sand castles near the dock, in her cute little green, string-top bathing suit that never quite covered her little bottom. One of the photo albums or one of the home movies had framed her forever in that green bathing suit, with a dart in her hand, tongue sticking out the side of her mouth in total concentration, ready to toss and hit the bull's-eye. Framed only in memory was the picture of Jeannie that same summer, with a sputtering sparkler in her hand, ready to celebrate the Fourth of July.

Larry was there to take Greg to watch the fireworks at the Fairgrounds. He asked his son, "Will it be cold? I left my cover—I mean my coat—in my bedroom."

"Okay, let's go get it. Do you want to take the stairs or the elevator?"

"The car."

"We can't drive upstairs, Dad."

"I know that! Not the car we drive; the car that goes up and down, the whaddayacallit."

"The elevator?"

"That's it."

1947

Fireworks! And the time they celebrated July 4ᵗʰ at the lake with their Canadian friends, for whom even an Independence Day that wasn't theirs was a great reason for a party. Larry had saved his allowance, had pestered and pleaded to be allowed to buy some of the fantastic fireworks for sale at tented tables conveniently located at the corner of every road just outside the Fargo city limits.

"I know Canadians don't celebrate the Fourth of July, but they wouldn't mind if we did, Dad, and all our friends would come to watch our rockets bursting over the lake. Everyone loves to watch fireworks. Please, Dad?"

And Greg remembered promising to think it over and secretly knowing he would agree, because he, too, wanted to see rockets over the lake.

To all the kids, impatiently asking, "Isn't it ever going to get dark?" and all the equally eager adults who hid their anticipation somewhat better, the ever-so-gradual darkening of the sky seemed to take forever. The afternoon's fitful breeze that hadn't quite raised whitecaps on the ruffled lake had died down, leaving the lake a sheet of dark glass. Another sunset, the kind that local and visiting artists tried fruitlessly to capture on canvas, had slowly faded away.

Finally, the dusk became dark, and off they trooped, down the gnarly tree root steps of the hill to the smooth, still sun-warmed sands of the beach. For an old lady, Mrs. B. scampered down the hill as adroitly as the kids. All the MacKenzie kids were there, and Judy and Bruce Ross, looking like Jack Spratt and his wife, and the Crawfords, kids and parents, and the Frankes and others whom Greg barely noticed, so intent on his job of fire master.

After Larry had equipped each child and all willing adults with sparklers, Greg lit his own and then touched the one nearest him and slowly an ever-widening ring of twinkling candles sputtered and fizzed in the quiet. From across the lake a loon called to its mate.

Then it was time for the big bangs. Greg carefully supervised while Larry anchored the first rocket, aiming it high over the waiting water, and lit it. Nothing. A soft swoosh. A faint light trail up into the sky, and then the explosion that made everyone jump before the chorus of "Ooohs" as the rocket novaed in a widening circle of crimson confetti.

Each successive rocket and blaster and banger seemed bigger and better than the one before until, at last, Greg launched the final four show stoppers simultaneously, and red, yellow, blue, and purple spheres merged and were reflected in the mirror of the lake, and it was over.

It was later that summer that Mother Nature quietly, proudly, breathtakingly filled the sky over the lake with her awesome answer to their little light show. Greg remembered that they had said goodnight to dinner guests and he'd gone for a head-clearing stroll along the lake shore. Looking above the forest on the opposite shore, he stubbed out his cigar and, no longer strolling, not quite running, went back to get his family.

Looking like all the veils of Salome, pastel ghosts were shape-shifting all across the northern sky—pale yellow merging into soft, faint green, replaced by a tissue the color of the mid-day sky, sliding into a haze of purple, then shadow-crimson. From east to west, horizon to zenith, the ripple of colors danced. He thought he could almost hear a sigh of melody. Gradually the colors faded until only murky white veils shimmered across the expanse of sky. And then it was dark. Holding hands, they came back to earth and went to bed.

It was hard to pull his thoughts out of that time, that place, those beloved people. When he did make the effort to return to the now, too often his only companions were the white coats and the remains of the once-alive, who slumped in armchairs and wheelchairs, ignoring the television that was always on and that no one watched, often with their mouths agape, sometimes drooling.

When the real-alive came, and smiled and hugged him, he tried, he really tried very hard to know what their mouths were saying and to make his mind and his mouth work together. He understood what their eyes were saying—they loved him and it hurt them.

Sometimes, for a rare minute, it all worked together—"Floy/Judie/Jeannie/Larry—I love you!" Mostly, only his eyes would let him talk. The names, the words, the thoughts went back into the storage boxes of his brain.

The pretty lady with the blue eyes like his brought a bouquet of flowers, the kind he remembered from a garden behind a house someone's mother lived in—his wife's mother, that was it. Peonies. He liked flowers. He especially liked wild flowers, the kind that grew like Topsy wherever they chose, but usually did not survive even the most gentle attempts at transplanting.

In the early years at the lake, regulations may have existed discouraging or forbidding digging up and relocating the park's wildflowers, but no one mentioned such regulations, if there were any, so Greg dug and transplanted to his heart's content.

Pine-sappy and stick-to-your-shoes loamy, the path from the back door and down the hill to the lake shore needed, Greg thought, boundaries. Otherwise, stray hikers and often children, his own and others, plodded or skipped across what was supposed to be the front lawn, a smallish patch of scrubby grass struggling to survive under the shadowy umbrella of the towering pines. Sunshine rarely penetrated.

Nature had provided steps down the hill—tree roots had pushed above ground, making an effective erosion barrier that also prevented people from suddenly slipping on the pine-needled surface and sliding down the entire slope right into the lake.

But Greg wanted to define the path from the cottage to the top of the hill. He lugged stones, deciding early on a size limit for his back's sake, and edged the path. He raided a gravel pile near the cottage but out of sight of neighbors or cruising Mounties, loading buckets to haul home in the trunk of the car. He spread the gravel the full length of the path, between the rock borders, refusing to count the number of trips he made with his buckets.

Time for flowers. A few coy violets hid under the few trees between his cottage and the rental one to the east, but lots of open space awaited adornment. Since the violets that were already there were thriving, surely moving more of the dainty things from deep in the woods where no one could enjoy them would not hurt. More trips with buckets, until there was a carpet of purple and green in the little forest.

He dug Indian paintbrush, and lovingly put the plants and what he thought was an ample supply of surrounding soil in an open, sunny area, since they seemed to prefer the open space of ditches along roads. After a half-dozen futile attempts at getting it to re-root and thrive, Greg decided that Indian paintbrush was vibrantly colorful growing wild, seen from a distance, but up close it was rather coarse, and smelled rank.

He then tried wild columbine. Its colors ranged from deep blue to dusky pink to a soft red-orange, more red than orange. Starting with just a few, he waited to see if they could successfully make the transition from out-in-the-country roadside ditch. No problem. Eventually, the path was columbined the entire length of the path, three to six feet wide.

Prairie roses were less successful, but clumps of them shared the earth with wild strawberries (so tiny; so sweet) all along the beach path, and a few stayed where he put them near the cottage.

Greg's favorites, and the kids', were the harebells (never called anything but bluebells—politically incorrect, but descriptive; they were blue, and they were elegantly fluted bells.)

Greg worked on his wildflower garden every summer: windflowers (Canadian anemone), wild phlox, butterwort, fringed milkwort, ferns (Jeannie said he fussed them too much; they grew better under her benign neglect), Solomon's seal, bastard toad flax (half the fun of his garden was sharing the names of his pet plants with guests), and—the crowning glory, yellow ladyslippers that decided they liked the sunny area where the larkspur were, near the porch windows.

He remembered someone giving him a book about Canadian wildflowers, pleasing him because it gave him the proper names of his treasures, but he hid it on a bottom shelf of an end table because the description of each floral gem included the warnings "These are rare —should only be picked or moved under special restrictions or permit," and "Do not pick or dig up." The warnings were too late to prevent what had already happened, but he didn't want some busybody thinking he'd deliberately flouted the law.

They had all offered to help, but this was his pleasure, not theirs. Floy cherished the shrubs and flowers around the yard in Fargo. She had poured over the designs submitted by the landscape companies, conferred with Greg about the best plan, and contentedly watched through the windows while each bush and bulb and seedling was bedded down in the exact spot dictated by the master plan. She rarely ventured off the lawn into the flower beds to pull a weed. She'd seen a snake once.

The kids were busy sleeping in or at the dock in their bathing suits, cavorting in and out of the water with their friends. They were too old—or too young—to enjoy grubbing around in the dirt.

And Greg enjoyed his own solitary company. Apart from the war years when he and Mike had done their business traveling together to stretch their gas coupons, he had spent a good part of every week day from September to June alone in his car, planning his day and mentally revisiting people and places from his past.

Transplanting each little contraband wildflower of the hundreds that eventually bedecked the sides of the path and the keep-out-the-neighbors flower bed along the front lawn, his hands and eyes worked with unconscious precision, needing no attention from his wandering thoughts. Greg's mornings in his evolving garden were between him and the One who, on the third day, had created flowers. Greg's family and his friends could have him the rest of the day.

He heard them talking, the old one to the young blond one: "He doesn't talk much anymore, dear, so don't expect any conversation, but he seems to listen and to understand what he hears."

He did listen and sometimes he did understand. He was listening very hard as she was describing how the flowers looked this year. The ladyslipper had kept going and had even transported part of itself several feet away. She. Jeannie? Yes—blue eyes, blond hair. His wife and other daughter had deep brown hair and eyes. His son was a hybrid—light brown hair, blue eyes.

10

A HOME OF THEIR OWN

On one of their drives around Fargo, Greg asked Jeannie if she would please go by his old home. He couldn't quite remember what it looked like; his mind seemed to have several images of "home," all different.

He remembered a small, tidy, two-story house on a small, tidy lot in a village surrounded by wheat and corn and potato fields. His mother and father and his brothers and sisters had moved from the little farmhouse out in the fields he loved into that small, tidy house in town. He was only five years old. He had loved the farm—the rich smell of a just-plowed field, the look of tiny seedlings as they suddenly popped out of the earth after a rain, the feel of the velvet noses of the horses.

His mother had said there would be lots of horses at the livery stable his father had traded the farm for, but Greg didn't want to leave the farm, and he didn't like the new house. It wasn't really new: it was older, smaller, and shabbier than his birth home.

Greg remembered another house, a country ranch house a couple miles from neighbors, in tree-and-rock-covered hills, where he used to take long walks every morning and get together with his and his wife's many friends in the late afternoons.

The house Jeannie drove him to was a big, beautiful, two-story white house on a large, meticulously landscaped lot, with a white picket fence in the back yard. It was the home his children had grown up in, a house someone else now lived in.

Greg remembered unlocking the front door and following Floy inside their new home. Their house. A brand new, never lived in by anyone before house. A house that smelled new—of fresh paint, sawdust, wallpaper paste, plaster, carpet—and looked new—pristine sinks and bathtub, fingerprintless woodwork, gleaming and scratchless stove and oven, spotless refrigerator, closet walls as yet unmarked by the scrape of hang-

ers. Even the furnace was mirror-bright. Greg could almost see again Floy's twirl around that bare living room, mentally arranging the furniture they didn't yet have.

"The couch will go there, with a coffee table, do you think? And over here, facing each other, easy chairs with separate end tables and good reading lamps. Oh, Greg, it is a dream!"

Her plans were almost perfect; he had only one addition: "Honey, do you think the dining room is spacious enough for a really long dining table and also a buffet? I like buffets."

Floy was agreeable: "I think so. Then the silverware and the table linens would be safely stored and also accessible." And twirling again, she exclaimed, "This is wonderful! We are homeowners!"

Greg agreed it was a wonderful house. And it wasn't a wonderful new house in a strange city; it was a wonderful new house in the city where they had gone to college, the city where many of their college friends still lived, the city where Mrs. B. was a short two blocks away. The children would finally get to know one of their grandmothers.

The grade school was only six blocks away, on safe streets for children walking there and back home every day. Downtown, there were department stores and hotels and restaurants and all the other trappings of a city.

And churches. Floy chose the First Presbyterian Church for Larry and Judie's religious education, not because she liked the minister—she didn't: he was a sour John Knox adherent, all hellfire and brimstone—but because she admired the elegant architecture, the lofty stone building that covered a whole city block.

Many Sunday mornings in the fall, after dropping the kids off at Sunday School, Floy and Greg returned home, Greg to load the car, Floy to busy herself with sandwich making—her renowned ground-up Spam, onions, and mayonnaise filling her equally renowned but more palatable baked-yesterday bread. Each half-sandwich was wrapped in a separate, carefully measured piece of waxed paper and then lovingly packed into the sandwich-sized metal box that, with two thermos bottles, composed the picnic set that went with them on all their trips. The red-capped thermos was for milk, the black-capped one for coffee.

Floy and Greg wore scruffy clothes. Floy, who normally wore slacks only for the grimiest household tasks, was outfitted in a pair of corduroy slacks so tired that the original color had long since been beaten out of them by repeated sessions in the washing machine with such company as the throw rug by the back door and saddle blankets from the farm.

Above the slacks were two sweaters that might have come from a Salvation Army refuse pile. Their once bright colors—red and orange—would have fought if they *hadn't been so faded. Greg wore ancient khaki pants and shirt. He couldn't remember if they had ever been new.*

He and his wife hadn't dressed for church; they weren't going to church. They were all going pheasant hunting. After Floy got the lunch ready, Greg loaded the picnic set into the car with the two shotguns, extra sweaters just in case, his and Larry's hunting coats—designed with numerous, ample-sized pockets for shotgun shells and a whistle, and clothes for the kids as disreputable as those he wore.

Then back to church to pick up the kids, who gleefully shed their Sunday School, dress-up outfits, trading them for clean but stained and somewhat tattered slacks and flannel shirts. They were off!

Off to a hunter's dream of a cornfield within an easy half hour's drive. Pheasants like cornfields. So do farmers, who were happy to have Sunday hunters reduce the overabundance of the pesky birds.

The next time Larry came, Greg told himself to remember to ask him how the pheasant population was this year. Back when the kids were little, the birds were so plentiful that the daily limit was six pheasants per hunter. But several hard winters had decimated the flocks, and Greg had stopped hunting when Larry went off to college and the limit dropped to one pheasant a day.

Greg remembered a conversation with an acquaintance who was virulently opposed to hunting. He respected the man's viewpoint, but was appalled at his ignorance. The guy had never hunted, but he seemed to assume that the pheasants lined up in open ground like bowling pins, and, helpless, were executed in vast numbers.

People like that had no understanding of the reality and were not willing to learn. Greg remembered hours spent tiptoeing quietly from one row of corn to the next, occasionally parting the stalks to peer into the next row, knowing full well that the pheasant he had seen not long after leaving the car was tiptoeing equally quietly one row over.

Once, when he parted the stalks to check the next row, he came face to face with a deer. They both jumped several feet in the air and whirled to get away from a marauder who should not have been there. It is impossible to see over or through a row of corn. Only the long alleyways between rows, stretching sometimes for half a mile, are visible. Pheasants know that. They are not stupid.

Greg did not disagree that cock pheasants are beautiful creatures, graceful in flight—and fast enough to outpace all but the most accurately aimed ammunition. Before he ever held a gun, before his first pheasant, he could identify a cock pheasant in flight.

Its head was a Technicolor target. The black skull cap might be effective camou-flage on the ground, but silhouetted against an azure sky, it simply drew the hunter's eye to the splash of scarlet around the eyes—the bull's eye. Not yet finished, Mother Nature had painted the entire neck a brilliant sapphire/turquoise/emerald, and con-cluded with a broad white ring at the base of the neck.

Greg's first kill both elated and saddened him. Until he held his still-warm bird, he had thought the body, as if compensating for the fatal brilliance of the head, was simply dull tan. Looking closely, he could see the tiny dots of blue and green, ringed by russet, that color in turn circled by a deep chocolate brown. Those "eyes" were scattered throughout the tan hues of the other body feathers.

Like all ethical hunters, Greg killed only what his family would eat—admitting that roasted pheasant was exquisite, and he could have bought a chicken. The point about hunting, Greg figured, was that it assured a balance—not so many pheasants that their wild food supply was inadequate and they were forced to forage in farmers' cornfields before a hard winter killed over-extended flocks too accustomed to the easy pickings of cultivated fields.

The wiliest pheasants, the survivors, especially the hens, whose drab brown attire rendered them invisible if they stayed earth-bound, wintered safely in berry-rich thick-ets and did not build their nests in flood plains.

◆　　◆　　◆

Jeannie, visiting for the weekend, inadvertently reminded him of one of the big Fargo floods. She asked why she hadn't been born at St. John's Hos-pital, as Larry and Judie had been, but at St. Luke's. He'd had to think back. Jeannie was born in the spring. Oh, yes, the year the Red River flooded not just Island Park, but the lower floors of St. John's, and the 20-acre hayfield across the street from their house, and the basement.

Floy was in the hospital for the ten days they used to keep new mothers and their babies. The saturated earth between First Street and the river soon was standing water on the lawn, and then it started seeping through the concrete walls of the base-ment, pooling and then rising until Larry asked if he and Judie could please go swim-ming.

Had Floy been there, the answer would have been an outraged "No!" However, the sewers hadn't backed up, the water that came up to his knees as he moved canned goods and spare toilet paper to higher perches was relatively clean, having been strained through the basement walls, and he had run out of ideas to keep the kids amused. So making them promise never, ever to tell their mother, he agreed to let them bring down a couple of bathtub toys—boats and a rubber duck—and go wading. They didn't stay very long—that water was frigid! Greg pretended he hadn't heard Larry ask if they could go fishing.

He remembered that Floy had asked the kids if they had behaved themselves while their dad was in charge. Both angelic faces nodded and said they'd done all their homework and read a couple books and helped Dad with the meals and keeping the house clean. Floy knew her children better than that, but she didn't pursue the matter.

Seeing the house where he and Floy and the kids had lived, loved, celebrated, and mourned before they had all scattered to Minnesota, Michigan, California, and Arizona, Greg remembered revisiting the village of his childhood.

He had not wanted to return to Lake Park ever again after his mother's funeral and burial. He didn't go for his father's. But more than 30 years after her death, alone on his way to see Larry and Barb, he turned off Highway 10 into the town. It was the same, but different, no longer looking downtrodden, worn out, too tired to fight back, growing smaller and smaller as kids like the boy he had been finished school and left for jobs, college, the "real world" and never came back.

It took a while for him to identify the difference—it looked like his boyhood memories, not the more recent ones, because all the houses and the shops, with "open" signs in their windows, looked prosperous with their fresh coats of paint.

His memory of the town the last time he'd seen it, the day of his mother's funeral, was of peeling paint —or none—on houses and boarded-up shops. People had been too poor for paint and too misery-sunk to wield a paint brush if there had been money for paint.

When he was a boy, it was a tidy, clean village with a very few expensive homes, but mostly modest ones. Until he left home for good, the area prospered; crops were bountiful and the town businesses were thriving, especially the new implement dealer, with shiny new tractors that were destined to replace farm horses. Some had forgotten, but those who watched the prosperity literally dry up and blow away never would.

The years of drought hit Alberta, the Dakotas, and the farmlands of Minnesota years earlier than the southern plains, and in those areas it lasted nearly two decades. The depression was bad, but the drought was worse. With no rain, dust storms that hid the sun, grasshopper plagues, and cutworms in summer and days-long blizzards in winter, the few farmers with anything to sell often paid more for seed than they got for their crops.

They went back to using horses, which they couldn't really afford to feed, because they couldn't afford gas for the tractors, many of which were repossessed for lack of payments. Businesses and banks, dependent on the farmers, closed.

Finally, in the late 1930s, the rains came. As the upper Midwest began recovering from the long years that had driven many farm families off their great-grandparents' farms, the war started. The few young men left in town went off to war; the few remaining young women took war-effort jobs in the cities. Their departure took what little spirit remained from those who stayed.

Greg's mother had died a year after the war started, and he had not been back to his boyhood home since her funeral. He had been appalled at the change, and had had no reason ever to revisit.

Ironically, it was partly thanks to the war that the area recovered; the entire national economy surged. The climate change helped, too, of course, but with a renewed demand for foodstuffs and decent prices for farm produce, the abandoned farms were swallowed up by huge conglomerates, with modern farming methods that would preserve the soil and trap the moisture instead of stripping it bare for the winds to ravish. And they had the money for big, mechanized equipment. The bankers and shopkeepers had a new clientele, and homeowners had both the pride and the paint to refurbish the town.

He had driven out to the Lutheran cemetery—this tiny town of just 700 people had three: one for Lutherans, one for Catholics, and another one for some other bunch. He'd taken flowers for his parents' graves. His mother had loved flowers; his dad wouldn't have cared.

But Greg had stopped despising his father. The man had dried out and stayed sober the last ten or fifteen years of his life. And Greg had felt the lure of liquor himself, to ease disappointment, to relax, to lighten up with friends, though he had been very careful to avoid excess.

Maybe it really was a disease, an inherited one. Larry had it bad, even after it ruined his health and forced his retirement before his fiftieth birthday. Maybe he drank in a futile attempt to stop regretting some of the choices he'd made.

Greg remembered those angry, anguished words: "I'll never be as good as you at anything!" He had tried to tell his son years before that he should not work for the same company, that he definitely should not work in the same state, that he absolutely should not build the home for his family out at the farm. To the school administrators who had been Greg's friends for thirty years and more, Larry would always be his father's boy, never an adult in his own right. Larry could make the friends he craved with new, young men, but never the old ones. He'd always be Greg's son, and, in his own mind, never as good at anything as his dad. Greg stopped showing his own horses when Larry started competing with his little herd, but he did not intend to retire for many years from the career he loved. Sadly, he understood that one can both hate and love one's idols. As a little boy, Greg had adored his own father. It had taken a lifetime to stop hating him.

He had resented his dad's never having time to play with him, or to go places with him. He did remember good times with Larry before he went away to college, and there had been amity between them after the bad years.

◆   ◆   ◆

"Take me out to the ballpark/Take me out to the game…" The lilting melody spread to the corner sofa where he sat with the nice boy—man? son? Yes, Larry. "You watch games," Greg announced, a memory surfacing for a time.

"Yes, Dad. Remember the Knothole Gang?"

He remembered a night when the kids had not returned at their usual ten o'clock, either gleeful that the Fargo-Moorhead Twins had won, or excusing their heroes' loss on the grounds of rotten pitching, blind umpires, or bad luck.

Before he and Floy began to imagine the worst—an explosion at the baseball park, a riot, a traffic accident—something that would render their children maimed for life—or worse yet, he turned on WDAY to get the play-by-play announcer. It was one of those games, the kind farm clubs endured too often: the score was tied at 12-12, and the eleventh inning had just started.

Leaving the radio on, they assured each other that the Knothole Gang was a good thing. For 25 cents for the season, kids under 16 could sit in a specially supervised section of the stands for all home games.

By 10:30, another inning was over, but the score was still tied: 15-15 now. At 11:00, Greg drove to the ballpark to collect his offspring. It was a school night after all. The cop monitoring the Knothole Gang section let him in, and he located Judie first, then Larry, each sitting with their own friends and pretending they didn't see each other. Not surprisingly, they didn't want to leave. "Daddy, can't we just wait until the end of this inning? The Twins are going to win!"

Against his better judgment, but rather enjoying the smell of popcorn and dust, the avid faces of a hundred kids, and the chatter from the players on the field mixing with the vendors' cries of "Get your hotdogs here! Popcorn! Cracker Jacks!" he sat down, "Just til the inning's over."

Finally, at 11:30, score still tied at the end of the seventeenth inning, thanks to bases-loaded home runs by each team, he insisted. His kids and three others who thought their moms might be getting mad piled into the car and left, leaving the game's final outcome up in the air.

The game on TV was still going. As usual, no one was watching. Larry inquired, "Did you ever see Roger Maris play the year he beat Babe Ruth's home run record?"

"I did. Sixty-one in '61. You and your sister went to school with that boy and his brother. Back then, coaches thought the brother was better."

Now where had that come from, Greg wondered. He hadn't talked about baseball or much of anything else for a long time. If he could think the words, and sometimes he couldn't, his mouth couldn't say them. He had forgotten so much. He remembered one other thing.

"Both boys left Fargo High and went to the Catholic high school. Some fuss with coaches."

Greg suddenly smiled, at a momentary image of a baseball game at Shanley High, this one played by the nuns, habit skirts hiked up, creating baggy bloomers, so they could run faster and avoid tripping.

He had arrived early for a meeting with Sister Agatha, the principal, and two members of the senior class, to look at samples for class rings and graduation announcements.

Sister Agatha had always put the fear of God in Greg. She had one of those faces he guessed people called "ascetic." He supposed that wannabe saints had to wear faces that looked long-suffering, pious, unforgiving, stern, and other-worldly all at the same time, but he always thought her pursed lips, frosty eyes, and frown were judging him, and finding him wanting.

This Sister Agatha, clutching a baseball bat that she obviously knew how to use, her tongue just poking out the side of her mouth, and an unholy glee lighting up her entire countenance, was another person altogether. She whacked the ball for a line drive deep into center field, into the shrubs along the convent wall, ran like a gazelle to third base, and stood on the bag, triumphant. Then she saw Greg watching.

Sister Agatha started to put on her pious-principal face, and then lost it. She started to smile. Greg started to laugh. Soon, they were both doubled over, hooting with laughter.

The meeting went very well.

11

WHO? WHERE? WHEN?

He should remember his son's name, this man who walked with such difficulty. He thought he remembered a time when this man was a boy who ran
with ease, on football fields, baseball diamonds, and basketball courts. He
always talked to Greg casually, as though he had seen him just yesterday and
would again tomorrow. "Hi, Dad, I'm going to take you to Pelican Lake
today, and we'll go out on the golf course."

The drive took them on a road he thought he remembered, but the lake
wasn't his lake; the cottage was nice but it wasn't the cottage he remembered. This one had no logs, and it was very modern, house-like, with too
many windows. The boat was weird, a flat floating platform with chairs and
a motor in the back with a dashboard in front like a car. Greg remembered
his boat, a sleek hull and a motor that had hand controls right on the side,
so powerful it raised the prow above the water when it went full speed.

1950
They went for a round-the-lake cruise on that boat, hugging the shore, stopping for
the picnic his wife had packed. There were home movies of that glorious day, his wife
and kids watching the water for loons and ducks and scanning the shoreline for maybe
a deer or a bear.

His wife and his kids. He couldn't remember their names, but their faces
were fixed firmly in his mind. His son. Yes, this man looked like his son, but
so old! Larry, that was his name. He was saying something—"Let's go meet
some friends for lunch and then go see the golf course."

He used to play golf every day on that magnificent course. So many of the holes gave
differing views of the lake that he forgot how much time was spent searching for errant
balls in the rough or in the woods.

The 17th hole was his favorite, even though he rarely managed par. He could see himself teeing up and looking down, down, down to the green far below, on the other side of that lovely, inviting, golf-ball magnet stream whose pine-bronzed water bubbled along through the trees on one side and that elusive green on the other. He remembered playing with a foursome of friends, while Floy played a round with their wives.

There were the names he sometimes lost—his wife, Floy; his son, Larry. If he concentrated on eyes and voices, he didn't get so confused. He had clear pictures in his head of his wife and his children, even if the names sometimes slipped away. But the three women and the man who were with him sometimes didn't match those pictures. Until he looked into their eyes. Until he heard their voices. This voice—his son's: "You and mom used to play golf almost every day, didn't you?"

Floy had a classic golf swing, although the ball never went very far. She was just too small for a power drive. Sometimes just the two of them played together, tallying similar scores because he lost penalty strokes for balls lost in the woods or that pretty little stream on the 17th hole. Her strokes didn't go far, but they went straight.

"Dad, we're just going to rent a golf cart and ride around the course today, and you can meet some of the guys I'm playing with tomorrow."

Golf carts. That's what killed the game. People used to walk the course, all eighteen holes, carrying their golf bags or, if they were old, pushing a little wheeled bag cart—but they still walked. This wasn't his golf course, his lake, his boat, his cottage. He wanted to go home. But when he tried to tell this man—yes, his son—that he wanted to go home now, the words weren't there.

◆　　◆　　◆

His son was here again, the old man, not the boy. Why would his mind and his mouth not come up with his name? It didn't matter—Greg enjoyed whatever breaks in the routine sameness were offered.

He listened intently to what was being said. "Dad, let's take a drive to the Hutterite chicken farm. I think you'll enjoy it. They live in a small religious community, like the Amish in many ways, and they raise the world's best chickens—completely free-range, no force-feeding, no prison-pens, no artificial anything, and they weigh about seven pounds each, almost like small turkeys."

1942–45

They'd raised chickens at the farm during the war. When Ken, his nephew, George's son, got rheumatic fever and was bed-ridden, Greg had offered the farmhouse to Ken and his cute city-bred wife Amy, if she could create a little income for her family with chickens. He would forever remember Amy, turning her head so as not to look while she wrung chickens' necks. And the twins—two years old, curly red hair, so identical even their mother had been known to put a band-aid on the wrong child's owie finger.

At first, the farm was just for enjoying the horses with the kids, but when Floy was faced with putting oleomargarine on the table, the farm had come into its own.

The place where they served meals here had margarine. Greg didn't like it, even though it was butter-colored.

War margarine was nasty white stuff—whiter than the lard his mother used for pie crust—that came in a cellophane bag and had a red pill in it. You were supposed to squeeze the red pill and keep squeezing until it mixed in with the white stuff, turning it yellow. It still tasted worse than lard. So he had bought a couple of milk cows for Amy to tend, and they had real butter and cream, and buttermilk, and wonderful milk, although Floy fussed because it wasn't pasteurized.

This was a nice farm. Some religious group, the man had said. Clean. Even the pigs were clean, and the baby pigs were…what was that word?

Greg didn't remember waking his kids up in the middle of the night, and he didn't remember driving out to the farm, but he clearly saw the ecstatic faces of his children, enraptured by the tiny, clean, pink, squealing baby pigs, lined up sucking noisily along their huge mother's side. He remembered saying not a word when the kids assumed these piglets would grow up to be big pet pigs on someone else's farm, never imagining that they were destined to become the bacon and pork chops of their own breakfasts and dinners.

He also hadn't told them that the delicious home-canned meat that made mouth-watering sandwiches one summer was from an elk that Dave Carter had shot the previous winter just outside the park. They loved elk—live ones that on rare occasions they'd seen on trips to the Lake Audy animal enclosure. All sightings of that huge herd were magic, but the first one was pure fantasy.

1948
The Robertsons, Lil and Frank and the kids—whiny Ann, older, blasé Cynthia, and adenoidal Lyle—were visiting in late August, so they'd gone, as they did with all visitors, to Lake Audy to see the bison herd, hopefully spot a bear or two, maybe see some deer. They'd gotten out of the car for a stretch before heading back to the cottage when they heard a never-before-heard whistling.

They all thought it was some rare bird, so they trooped off into the woods, each child's hand in the clasp of an adult's (in case of bears). They followed the whistles, finding the walk itself a wild-flower-lover's delight, and they were following a game trail, so they weren't plowing through thorn thickets or wading through waist-high grasses and shrubs. They climbed a gentle hill overlooking a meadow ringed with birch and evergreen trees.

And there was the source of the whistling. Not birds, but a meadow filled with elk. Proud, antlered bulls and flirty catch-me-if-you-can cows—there must have been at least two hundred.

They stood as quietly as if the world had stopped breathing for a minute. The elk napped, nuzzled grass shoots, the bulls sidling up to the seemingly-reluctant cows, the sentinel—antlers and ears alert—crouched but not really lying down. For a gift-from-God moment, no one moved. Then a stray scent from the human invaders snapped up the sentinel's head, and within seconds, the entire herd melted into the forest.

For a moment, Greg wondered if dying was like that—just melting into another part of the universe.

◆　　　◆　　　◆

He seemed to be spending a lot of time sleeping. That nice lady in the white coat woke him up to tell him that the kids had all phoned, terribly disappointed, but airports were closed thanks to a blizzard blanketing most of the central U.S.

1944
Usually it was he who was away from home when a blizzard hit, since that so often happened in the middle of the week. But he remembered one Sunday when the snow began cascading heavily about noon and the wind started howling by mid-after-

noon, so by nightfall, the state was blanketed in up to 36" of snow, schools were closed statewide, and people were advised to stay where they were, off the roads.

That Monday was a rare gift—a day off, no place that needed going to, home with his wife and kids and a whole backyard of snow waiting to be shaped into forts and tunnels. Floy opted to stay indoors; Jeannie was too little: she could get lost in those snowdrifts. Floy preferred to spend the chance holiday cooking a pot of soup and a special dinner. Greg and Larry and Judie donned long underwear, two pair of socks, mufflers, warm stocking caps made by Grandma B., snowsuits, boots, and mittens, and they headed out into the storm—only as far as the back yard.

Greg stomped a path a few feet inside the fence to mark the construction site and then they all got to work. The snow was just about right for shaping into blocks that could be piled to make tunnel walls, and even, after a few failures when the whole attempt crashed onto their heads, the roof for the fort. This snow was perfect for packing hard and staying where it was put.

By lunchtime, when none of them could feel finger and toe tips, and when, for all of them, the areas between their mitten cuffs and jacket sleeves that always seem to bare themselves to the elements were chafed and cold, they were ready for soup.

Blast this blizzard! They told him that his kids' plans to spend Thanksgiving with him had to be cancelled. His wife had phoned, too. She said she would come later. The hotel staff assured him that there would be a delicious Thanksgiving dinner in the dining room. He didn't care about the food; Thanksgiving was family, all gathered to give thanks that they were together again. At least his wife would be there, and it wouldn't be the first Thanksgiving they'd spent by themselves.

1952

There was a blizzard that Thanksgiving, too, but early on, he and Floy had piled themselves and the 25-pound turkey she'd roasted the day before into the car. They planned to outrun the storm and get to Northfield before it hit. Normally his wife would have gently suggested that he not drive so fast, but this time, she kept peering at the odometer and sighing, "Good, we'll make it."

The two older kids were both away at college—the same college, which was nice, and had only the one day without classes, so if they couldn't get home, their parents and the turkey would come to them. Jeannie and Mrs. B were sharing their holiday together quite contentedly at home.

As they passed the city limits, the storm was blowing into their tailpipe, but they made it to Judie's dorm where it looked like the entire student body was waiting for them. Many hands lovingly lifted the turkey roaster out of the car, amid a chorus of thank yous, and after all but two young people had paraded after the food, Judie and Larry were there with huge smiles and hugs.

By the time they all got to the lounge, the other kids had arrayed a table with bags of rolls, plates of butter, jars of Miracle Whip, a can (opened already) each of cranberry sauce, black and green olives, pickles, and even a couple heads of lettuce. One brawny young football player, by the looks of him, was wielding a carving knife as if he had had practice. An hour later, the turkey was reduced to bones, some still being gnawed by stuffed students, the kitchen had miraculously produced pumpkin pie and whipped cream, and the only sounds to be heard were contented murmurs.

Greg and Floy had not slept in a dorm room for years, and they had never shared a dorm bed intended for a single student. The only choice was to cuddle. A wonderful holiday.

They weren't cuddling, but at least Floy was with him for this childless, friendless Thanksgiving. She tried to cheer him up: "Greg, you're not eating. I know you like turkey. It's too bad the kids couldn't come today, but they will again soon. Do eat your turkey."

Greg thought it was a sad excuse for a turkey, those skinny slices of overdone white meat; His wife knew he preferred dark. She would remember their first really big turkey.

Like the pennies, this came in a box from his boss—a huge box that the kids used as a fort, a plane, a Flash Gordon space ship for weeks until it finally disintegrated. Neither he nor Floy had ever seen a turkey that big except flapping around stupidly in a farmyard, unaware of its fate.

This one was all pinky-white and clean, ready to be stuffed with bread and onions and spices and baked. He remembered driving his little daughter to the railroad station to collect the annual box encasing the holiday turkey. And he remembered his wife diligently wielding her eyebrow tweezers on the pinfeathers. They had to go out and buy a roaster big enough for it to fit in. The oven barely held it. They ate turkey for days—with leftover potatoes and pie, in sandwiches, even tried it with an egg for breakfast—once. And they invited friends to share. Thankful indeed for turkey and good friends and children and work.

He was not thankful for the storm that spoiled this Thanksgiving. But surely the kids would be home for Christmas.

12

Time Like a River

He did not want to be here. Sometimes he could go some other where, some other when, just by thinking. He preferred the comfortable, exciting, happy places and times to the sad or frightening ones, but any where and any when were at least different. Here was always the same. Same food—minor variations between one meal and the next. Same chair, although the place was full of chairs, some occupied, some not, all equally devoid of conversation. Same wallpaper, same carpet, same bustling white coats, same immobile human relics.

Even never knowing to what place and time his thinking would lead him was a welcome break from sameness. He couldn't just order up memories. They had a schedule of their own, independent of any hope he had of keeping them in order. He remembered knowing once, because it was in a book, that past, present, and future were not separate blocks of time, but more like a river that rushes ahead for a while, eager to see what's ahead; turns back on itself and circles, like a fox seeking a gone-to-ground rabbit; then pokes along lollygagging, a child in no hurry to get to school; and sometimes returns to its origin, only to flow forward again.

A few people could nudge his thoughts into particular wheres and whens. Who they were seemed to hover at the edge of a curtain. Rarely, the curtain opened. That nicely dressed old lady with ruler-straight posture and confident step had only to say two or three words and he was transported. Wherever he was, whenever it was, was unimportant. Floy was there.

Two younger ladies who usually came separately—one blue-eyed, one brown—had only to hug him and he didn't have to understand the words to know a daughter was saying "Daddy, I love you."

And the man—so changed, shuffling, not striding—smiled, not just with mouth, but the entire face, especially the eyes. And yet there was pain in his son's smile. It had occurred to him that it hurt them to be with him.

His son stayed to have lunch with him, said he had a surprise. Instead of the usual green Jell-o with bits of canned fruit stuck in it for dessert, the serving girl brought a cake with numbers on it—the numbers eight and five, they told him, because it was his birthday.

And there were cards—cards with pictures and messages they read to him: "Happy Birthday, Dad," "Happy Birthday, Daddy," "Happy Birthday, Grandpa." One of the grandpa ones was signed, "Love, your Snookie Poo."

1960–65

He remembered Snookie Poo as a bald infant, then a toddler, then a nursery schooler modeling her mom's snow boots. He saw her every Saturday, not long enough to watch her attempts to feed herself, to enjoy her bath splashes, to sit on his lap or snuggle in his arms to watch birds, but for her first five years, he charted the week-by-week changes. Her mom, his daughter, had been his secretary, so every Saturday, he took his order books, receipts, and schedule to her house so they could keep his correspondence, check book, and tax data in order. Wendy loved her grandpa and showed it by playing quietly while he and her mom were working, just waiting for the signal, "Where's my Snookie Poo?" to come running for a cuddle.

He had seen her recently, hadn't he? With a little blond girl—her daughter, she said. He recognized his Snookie Poo, even all grown up. He didn't remember if he'd ever met her husband. He remembered seeing pictures of the wedding.

1934

He wasn't in this picture. Even if this was a dream, he'd always been in the pictures of his dreams. But he wasn't in this picture. Everyone else was there: his parents; his brothers and sisters all grown up but young, with wives and husbands and children, both big and small. Not quite everyone—Floy wasn't there; she was never comfortable around his parents. Mabel wasn't in the picture, and George wasn't, either, although George's wife was, looking sad, and his son Ken. Because Mabel and George were dead? But so was his mother, and she was in the picture, still beautiful at nearly 70.

He still missed his mother. He had missed her for more than forty years.

He knew the white coats were drugging him, to turn him into another their collection of the undead. He could now appreciate the gift of unexpected, quickly-finished dying. He could even feel grateful that his mother had never had to suffer the indignities of having to have her diapers changed by a coolly efficient nurse in a coolly efficient nursing home.

1943

His mother had fallen, breaking her hip. Obert had phoned—could Greg pick up him and Anna for the drive to the Minneapolis hospital? She needed an operation. Greg did not ask Floy if she would go with him. She might have said yes, because she loved him, but she did not love most of his family.

Greg's mind understood Floy's antipathy toward his mother; his heart didn't. Floy saw Johanna as a woman who didn't control her children, couldn't control her husband, and thought she was doing the right thing by not standing in their way. Floy had to believe she was in control of her world, her children, her husband. For her, loving required controlling. For Johanna, loving was letting go.

Greg hoped that for him and his brothers and sisters, loving their mother would not demand letting her go; not just yet. Hylda and Louie were already at the hospital; they lived only a few miles from the hospital. Rosella and her husband couldn't be reached. Eddie and Harriet were checking flights from the west coast.

The family waited, talking softly. The hospital waiting room seemed to require more quiet than a funeral parlor. Greg wondered if there was some universal hospital rule that dictated the décor of waiting rooms. They were uniformly drab and depressing. He asked Obert if he'd seen a sign over the door to this one, "Abandon hope all ye who enter here." Obert smiled sadly and agreed that he wouldn't be surprised if there were.

The carpet was that cold olive drab on which no spill of coffee or blood would show, with a harsh, thin pile designed to withstand the tromp of millions of feet without wearing out and to abrade the knees of those who prayed. The walls were a lighter shade of that same uncaring, impersonal, mood-lowering blah beige, with a stipple effect intended to camouflage the fingerprints of those who had nothing else to hold onto.

There were pictures on the wall—of shipwrecks on storm-tossed beaches with lurking, malevolent clouds above. One in particular looked like the paint-by-numbers picture one of the kids had done one summer.

Tables and chairs fit right in. Functional, if the purpose was to ensure that no one would get comfortable and doze off. Scratchy or slippery fabrics in more shades of brown—dark, like twice-used coffee grounds. The most recent magazine was a two-year-old <u>Mechanics Illustrated</u>.

They waited, talking in whispers, but longing to shout, to wake the dead, to wake the living before it was too late. Finally, the surgeon came: the surgery had gone well; he expected a full recovery, despite Johanna's age.

Greg phoned Eddie to tell him, and agreed when his brother said they'd wait and come for a visit within the month. Hylda told them all to come to her house for the night—plenty of beds. They were all back the next day, taking turns during visiting hours to sit with their mother. She looked good, a bit pale, said she was terribly tired.

The demands of Obert's farm and Greg's schedule nudged them into leaving after another day of keeping their mother company, even if she did sleep most of the time. The doctor assured them she'd be fine, ready soon to leave the hospital and go to Hylda's, where she would be well cared for.

Greg had been home only a day when Hylda phoned with the message he never wanted to hear, didn't expect to hear for many years: his mother was dead. Floy saw the appalled look on his face, and just held out her arms, holding him to her breast, saying only, "I am so sorry." He knew her sorrow was for him, not herself. She would not grieve the death of a woman she never really knew, never really wanted to know. Holding Greg in his grief was a precious gift. Floy then got very busy in the kitchen out of sight; she always had difficulty coping with emotions, her own or anyone else's.

Greg sat in stunned, silent grief on the couch, unheeded tears streaming down his face. His coltish daughter sat beside him with a box of Kleenex and silently held his hand, silently weeping—for him, not herself. She had met that grandmother only once in her life, when she was five years old.

So if he wasn't in the anniversary picture, was he dead, too? No. Now he remembered: he got there too late for the picture, but not for the party to celebrate his parents' fiftieth wedding anniversary. They looked young. His father even looked sober.

His sister Rosella was there, still the acid-tongued, stunningly lovely girl she'd always been. She was another reason Floy wouldn't have come: Larry was still in diapers and Floy was pregnant with Judie when Rosella smirked, "Looks like Greg has a brood mare." Floy never spoke to Rose again. Jeannie was not born until nearly nine years later.

Greg regretted that there were no pictures of his mother with his children. Everyone else's kids were in the anniversary photograph; his children were home with Floy that day. At home, there were boxes and albums full of pictures, even several reels of motion pictures. There were baby pictures and birthday party pictures and pictures of kids on horses. There were pictures of kids on the dock, jumping off the dock, being pushed off the dock. Graduation pictures, wedding pictures, grandchildren's baby pictures.

He must remember to ask the girls where all those pictures were, the snapshots and the home movies they'd watched so many times after renting the projector and the screen from the Osco Drug Store. Odd how long-forgotten, unimportant names and places briefly visited his memories and then vanished again.

Maybe the doctor would give one of the girls a prescription to take to that store for him. He was so tired. And so sick. His brown-eyed child whose one eye didn't always follow the other one seemed to know he didn't feel like listening and couldn't talk so she'd understand. She put her arm around him and let his head rest on her shoulder. She held him to sleep.

September 1991–June 1992
Nursing Home: Fifth Year

"Scraps of ideas flit like birds."
—Thomas DeBaggio

13

Nightmares and Fairy Tales

He was in the middle of a bad dream. At least he thought it was a dream, but he wasn't sure.

1949

He was driving, had been driving for hours. His wife and children and his wife's mother were with him, so he was more concerned than he would have been if he only had to worry about his own safety. The maximum speed he could achieve was fifteen miles an hour, because the road under his tires was a quagmire of deep, slippery, shifting sand.

Clenching the wheel, he tried to keep going in a straight line, but was forced, time and again, to go around one yellow behemoth after another—highway construction equipment. And it was hard to see. It was that time after sunset in June when twilight lasts for an hour or more, longer if one is heading north, as they were. The dim dusk sky was further blurred by billions of suspended grains of sand, stirred up by all the vehicles, filming the windshield.

They had always left for the lake by eight or nine in the morning. This time, Larry had something he had to finish before they could leave, so it was afternoon before they were on the road. Normally, they were at the lake in time for dinner, but this time, they'd had to stop in Dunseith to stifle the growly stomachs and whining kids. So they got to the construction zone just after sunset, and read with dismay the sign "Construction next 25 miles. Drive slow."

At some point in that nightmare trip, they crossed into Canada, but barely noticed when the border people waved them on through after a very brief exchange through the rolled-down window. Greg never remembered the rest of that trip; he guessed the car found its way to the lake once it got away from the cloying sand.

That dream kept coming back—he couldn't see clearly; he couldn't hear well; he couldn't talk; he was endlessly mired in sand, trying unsuccessfully to get back on a smooth highway.

Sometimes he wasn't just dreaming of past events, he was reliving them. Many were pleasant; a few were funny; some were disquieting.

1949

Greg liked to walk along the beach to Deep Bay. Often he took off his socks and shoes—they were going to fill up with sand anyway, and he liked the feel of soft, warm sand squishing through his toes. Some childhood pleasures never go away.

During the war, it was called Airplane Bay: it housed a small Canadian Air Force post where pilots practiced seaplane take-offs and landings before the troops and the planes headed for Europe.

As he reached the point that marked the start of the bay, the usually empty dock was crowded with uniformed men and diving equipment. Curious, he drew close enough to say, "Good morning; may I ask what you're diving for?" knowing that the odd sunken rowboat or Jean Smith's speedboat motor were not important enough for a diving crew.

"Good morning, sir. You may have heard about the fisherman whose empty boat was found floating by the golf course?" Greg nodded. "Well, we assume he fell over-board, and the body has not yet been recovered. We think the boat drifted from some-place close to here. If he's under a rock shelf down 100 feet or more, he could stay there forever. If he doesn't show up, his wife would have to wait seven years before he's declared dead. So we're looking."

Greg was curious; he had to ask one of the divers, "What's it like down there?"

"It is another world, an incredibly beautiful world" was the reply. "If you've seen mountains?" Greg nodded. "Well, imagine low mountains, hills really, with over-hanging ridges of rock, in soft, subdued colors—tans, grays, russets, blacks, mossy greens, a bit of blue—and curious fish darting in and out and coming up to your face to check you out."

Thinking of the serenity and the alien beauty of a cave under the waves, Greg thought it would be a nicer grave than some he had seen. He hoped the man's wife could come to realize that, to hope the body would never surface, to pray she could remember him as he looked when she saw him last. After a week or more immersed in water, the body would trigger nightmares.

Greg avoided Deep Bay for several days, returning only when he saw in the news-paper that the man's body had been found, the funeral held, the far away grave marked.

Deep Bay had become the graveyard of the once proud motor launches that had carried hundreds of sightseers, thirty at a time, on tours around the lake, twice a day for several years until speedboats and water skiers drove them away. There were four of them, now beached forever at what was once their winter quarters. Traces of the once jaunty blue and white paint still stuck to the rotting boards. Not enough of the black script formerly announcing the name of each launch remained for him to pick out the names he had forgotten.

Greg had taken Floy and the kids on the round-the-lake launch trip once. They'd all had a delightful time—perhaps not so delightful for the other passengers, since the kids kept pointing out the barely seen glimmer of white that marked the Purvis' cottage, the frankly garish yellow and green of the MacMorran's, and several log cottages—visible only if you knew they were there, and indistinguishable unless you knew the lake and its people very well, They did. Tourists on a week or two holiday did not, and very likely did not care.

Deep Bay slumbered for years, the old launches sinking further and further into the sand, the once-broad beach path to the sentinel point washed away during years of high water, leaving a scattering of sand overwhelmed by rocks. Then the water skiers discovered it. Although no one could stroll on sand to get to the bay, it was easily accessed by boat and, a little less easily, down the stairway from the parking area on Wasagaming Drive.

The abandoned launches how had the company of dozens of fast, noisy, crayon-hued boats, berthed in the bay all summer and swarmed during the day by skimpily-clad young people with their water skis and surfboards. And their radios, each blasting a different pop tune. Once, Greg heard the melody of "Try to Remember."

Those speed boats could run at idle in 80–100 feet of water, two or three feet from shore, where the skier, feet in the rubber stirrups, hands on the rope attached to the boat, gave the signal and the boat was put into high gear. If the skier fell, it was into the cushion of deep water, not the abrasive, not-very-yielding sand of the beach.

Water skiing at Deep Bay was safe, but young people don't seem to understand the word. Indelibly etched on Greg's brain was the slow-motion picture of his son behind a speed boat on his water skis, holding the rope with one hand and waving to his family and friends on the dock with the other, while his friend Gus aimed the boat at the dock and veered off. Gus either forgot or didn't realize that the skier's arc would be wider than the boat's. As Larry sped inexorably toward the dock, doomed to crash into the boards that were built to withstand the icebergs that formed when the ice went out of the lake, Greg saw his son's deeply tanned face turn white and his broad grin fade into a rictus of sheer terror.

Somehow, instinct kicked in, and Larry let go of the rope. The horrified, helpless audience on the dock watched as the skis and skier, slowly—agonizingly slowly—started to sink Greg's last sight before he remembered to breathe again was his son's face disappearing safely under the jutting boards of the dock.

Thinking about Deep Bay, Greg remembered another day, a day starting in panic and ending in contentment.

1941

Pray God and all His angels that the child had not gone to Deep Bay. He and Floy had just returned from the golf course. The carpenter's daughter who was supposed to be tending the kids had again spent her time baking incredible pastries in the wood stove's oven. Perhaps the girl wasn't old enough for the responsibility, but dagnabbit! his children were more important than Danish pastries.

The boy could be heard, playing cowboys and Indians in the nearby woods. He didn't know where his little sister was. He'd got tired of her joining all his games and told her to go away.

She loved taking walks along the shore to Deep Bay, but always with an adult. She wasn't quite seven years old. Could she have gone there by herself? Would she have?

All along the shore to the point that marked the start of Deep Bay, it was shallow enough for a child to wade for the first several feet, and then it deepened slowly. But around that point, the soft broad sandy beach beckoned the unwary into the water where, two feet from shore, it dropped off to a depth of 80–100 feet. Joan Smith's outboard motor could still be seen there, where it had fallen after she'd forgotten to fasten it to the boat before trying to start it. Show-offs would dive from the sand into the depths.

The child could dog paddle, but she hadn't yet learned to hold her breath and wait for clear air before inhaling. Surely she would remember the danger and not go wading.

He remembered nothing of the run along the shore and around the point. He remembered forever the heart-stopping sight of his little daughter serenely building a sand castle, several feet from the treacherous water. He wanted to snatch her up and shake her until her teeth rattled, He wanted to hug her breathless. He smiled at her joyful face and said, "It's time to go home, honey." And they walked along the friendly lake shore, holding hands, discussing dinner possibilities and bedtime stories.

Did he still tell the children bedtime stories? He couldn't remember, but it seemed a long time since he had done that. Maybe "Goldilocks and the Three Bears" needed to be revised again, to keep it fresh.

He'd started embellishing the tale one evening after a supper of split pea soup and homemade bread. The kids had griped about oatmeal for a long time, dutifully eating the lumpy glop for breakfast two or three times a week, but always asking to have it disguised under generous spoonsful of brown sugar or chopped dates. They had never believed any self-respecting bear or golden-haired fairy tale heroine would eagerly consume the stuff. They knew that "porridge" and "gruel" were just other names for oatmeal. Different names did not make the reality any better and it could hardly be worse.

Maybe it was the split pea soup, maybe it was his chopping a bit of kindling for the fireplace before supper, maybe it was a fleeting memory of the rhyme "Pease porridge hot, pease porridge cold..." that pricked his imagination. That evening, the embellishments began, with Papa Bear at the chopping block, splitting the peas for the dinner soup. Now there was an acceptable motive for Goldilocks to taste all three bowls and not to flinch at the "too hot," nor gag at the "too cold," and then to scrape the bottom of the "just right" bowl. And now it was perfectly understandable that the bears were outraged that their dinner had been tampered with.

He also changed the end of the story, tossing in a suitable moral about good manners: the bears invited Goldilocks to stay and have supper with them, and she graciously accepted. Had it been oatmeal, not pea soup, she could be excused for running away screaming.

Oatmeal was served here for breakfast. Before he moved here, he had always fixed his own breakfasts of two fried eggs, two rashers of bacon, and two pieces of toast, along with orange juice and coffee. Other food here was okay, apart from the meatloaf. And he always looked carefully at the salads, but never found dandelion greens. He didn't care for them. He didn't know anyone except his wife that did.

1941

"My throat hurts. I can't eat this salad; it scratches. Can we have ice cream?" This was getting out of hand, but who wants to call their children liars? Con artists, yes. They had stopped in Minot for a few days on their way to the lake to have the kids' tonsils out. The doctor had said they would have sore throats for a while and could be pampered a bit with Jell-o and ice cream.

But it had been a month now, and surely their throats were healed? They managed to eat other scratchy foods—crisp bacon, roasted peanuts, raw carrots and celery, dill pickles, and potato skins slathered with butter. Their faces when they saw their mother picking dandelion greens for the dinner salad should have warned him that tonight was going to be another sore throat night. He didn't much like dandelion greens, either, but his generation had learned early that you ate everything on your plate, like it or not, because that's all there was.

Memories of insignificant events he had thought to be long vanished were surfacing more and more often these days. He wondered why. He felt rather comforted: some of the husks of humans strapped in their wheel chairs near him did not seem to have memories—or minds. Their eyes, "windows of the soul" someone had called them, were blank, unfocussed. These creatures didn't move. Couldn't? He still went for walks, but walks were afternoon things.

After breakfast and after dinner he didn't want company. He went back to bed. Shirley—no, she was gone. Now it was JoAnn; wasn't that his mother's name? No, hers was Johanna—it was JoAnn who kept him company in the afternoons and would sometimes walk with him. His son came, too, but he now had trouble walking, so mostly they drove to places he didn't recognize and feared he had forgotten.

14

HE USED TO KNOW THEM

Living and reliving in other whens became nows. She and He and They broke in at times. Living and reliving was easy; fitting the bits together, terribly hard. She had come to join him for dinner.

They were in the elegance of his dining room at Mooswa and all the girls in their cute uniforms had come over one at a time to say "Good evening, Mr. G," "Good to see you, Mr. G." and their own girl knew without asking that he wanted crumbled blue cheese on his salad with French dressing, and that he'd ask for a bottle of Jordan Valley sparkling red wine with dinner. Most of the guests were tourists and he didn't know them and they didn't know that he owned this place and he didn't tell them, but the summer residents who came there for dinner were all long-time friends. It was nice there.

The words weren't uttered. He smiled at her. She suggested "Let's take a drive."

They turned left out of the driveway and took the lakeshore drive, going straight where a left turn would have taken them to the golf course, and went onto the Norgate road. The fire that everyone had feared would destroy the park just cleansed it. Wildflowers were everywhere—he wanted to ask her to stop so he could dig some to transplant at the cottage, but said nothing. One time when they were here, they had passed a young moose, standing right by the side of the road, staring as hard at them as they were at him. Backing the car up to take a picture sent him disappearing in an eyeblink into the woods. No picture, except forever in memory.

After they got to the top, unaware that the car had been straining uphill all the time, they always got out of the car and climbed the ladder of the observation tower to survey the tiny toy town miles below in the mists of the vast, faraway plain. Turning the car around, he always put it in neutral, turned off the engine, and started coast-

ing. He could still hear the kids' countdown: "Four point one...four point five...four point seven...four point eight! One of these days we'll do five miles!" They always hit a straight stretch that slowed the car to a crawl before they got to the magic number. Someone had told him cars can't do that anymore.

"Wake up, dad—we're back."
Would he ever be truly back?
"Would you like to sit outside for a while? Let's go sit over there, in the sun."

He remembered afternoons sitting on the dock. The MacKenzies or at least most of the kids—never the parents—were always there: the red headed freckle-faced friend of Larry's, the older blond who looked like a linebacker, the skinny one that died of leukemia, and the dark-haired handsome one—Ray, who married Beth Crawford. Good friends. There were MacKenzie girls, too—Kay who wasn't pretty but very kind, Lorna who was elegant and—once you got to know her—very funny, and another one whose name he didn't think he'd ever known.

The kid who had been so badly stung by wasps that time was there, as were the little Rickett kids, building sandcastles with Jeannie.

He had seen Barb and Rick recently, he thought. Spunky Barb, ready for a party, a golf game, a happy hour, relieved that her children were now old enough to go to the dock by themselves to meet Jeannie and the rest of their friends and sip their Bloody Marys. (They thought their parents really believed the thermoses were full of iced tea. Parents are not stupid.)

Barb was not herself. Floy had told him that she had been diagnosed with Parkinson's disease, but he hadn't realized that she would be a skinny, tremor-ridden travesty of herself. If she had not had a tight grip on her cane, and Rick hadn't had a tight grip on her, she would have fallen on her walk down the driveway.

They had gratefully accepted the invitation to come in for a chat and a drink. Barb opted for water—no more G & Ts: her medications barred booze. There was nothing wrong with her mind. She was still full of kind gossip concerning lake people they knew and knew about. She was upbeat and cheerful, and funny, but Greg could see the effort it cost her.

Brash Rick, the cool Brit with the wry sense of humor, never solicitous of anyone, always chatty, now hovered around his wife, silent, letting her enjoy friends while she could.

Greg wondered which was worse, losing your mind while your body stayed robust, or continuing to be mentally acute while watching your body die.

Greg's lady looked at him as if she had been waiting for a response. He looked a question at her. "Barb Ricketts died, Greg. Remember Barb and Rick, our friends at the lake?" Barb who? he thought; I think I knew her. The lady looked sad, so he guessed he should, too, but if he had ever believed death was sad, he knew now that it was living and dying that were sometimes devastating, not death. Death was a release, a relief.

Barb had relieved the slight tension by reminding them all of the summer her friend Peggy had come for a week's visit, bringing her puppy. The puppy had turned out to be a vicious brute, an enormous, 18-month old Great Dane that considered all humans except his owner as potential attackers, and heeded not one word his mistress said. The Ricketts had spent the entire week afraid to enter their own cottage until assured that Tiny was shut in a bedroom.

Barb and Rick had previously invited their friends to a cocktail party to met Peggy, and either they hadn't warned their guests about Tiny or Greg and Floy had forgotten. They had approached the door, knocked once, and Greg was reaching for he doorknob when the entire screen door frame was filled with a slavering, snarling beast, upright with front paws clawing the fragile screen, daring them to move. Peggy appeared—half the size of her dog—coaxing, "Tiny, get down; Tiny, come here." Only when she grabbed his studded collar and whacked him on the nose did her reluctantly back off from his prey. The cocktail party conversation was punctuated by growls and heavy thumps from a closed bedroom.

Telling the story years after the fright, Barb thought it was hilarious, but Greg remembered that Peggy had not ever been invited back.

◆   ◆   ◆

Maybe all those friends would be at the lake this year, now that the war was over. He could visualize their faces, sometimes looking older than other times, but he knew them. He didn't know most of the people sitting near him in the sunshine. He wondered if he used to know them. They didn't seem to know him—just as well: he'd soiled himself.

He was mortified. He tried to remember if he had been sick, but he didn't think so. He was afraid he had forgotten that he needed a bathroom. The calm acceptance of the mess by the white coats somehow made him feel even worse, and when they put a huge diaper on him after they'd cleaned him up and got out clean clothing, he wept. And then he forgot that he hadn't always worn padding under his shorts. Sometimes he thought he smelled bad, but visitors didn't seem to notice—or maybe they were too polite to say.

The man who had created the fireplace at the cottage was still a frequent visitor; he was here again with his friend. "Hey, Greg, dija hear about Ole's fishing trip?" Probably not—Curly rarely repeated his stories. Even if he had, Greg would have forgotten it.

Greg had never done much fishing. Never saw much joy in sitting on a hard boat seat getting sunburned, waiting for a random nibble. And neither he nor Floy ate fish if they could help it. But there was that one time.

1970

The Willoughbys had talked them into a fishing trip near Cranberry Portage, a famous fishing area in northern Manitoba. They made it sound like such a rare adventure that, to the surprise of everyone, Floy told Greg she would like to go.

They had a splendiferous time. Floy seemed to have forgotten that boats terrified her; ocean liners were the smallest water craft she normally would brave. But there they were, in a boat in the middle of a lake, actually catching fish—lots of fish. The open air and exercise awakened hunger pangs, and it was either that or the fact that the morning's catch of walleyes was so fresh that made their shore lunch one of the best feasts they'd ever savored.

Their guide tied up the boat on a small island and immediately got a fire going. The first priority was coffee. He piled rocks around the fire with a big flat one in the middle for the most disreputable coffee pot Greg had ever seen. Into that dented rusty pot the guide scooped water from the lake and waited for it to boil, setting out tin plates and cutlery and a roll of paper towels while waiting. Then he pulled a paper poke out of a cooler, dug out a handful of coffee and dumped it in the pot.

Next, the fish. They all watched in admiration as the guide laid a fish on a paddle, skinned it, filleted it, and laid it in a big, tatty-looking frying pan previously set on the fire with a blob of bacon grease scooped from a plastic container Greg hoped had not previously been used for worms. Onto the next fish. In less than 10 minutes, there were 20 fillets, some already out of the frying pan and onto plates.

The cooler yielded potato salad and cans of fruit cocktail, perfect accompaniments for those exquisite, crispy-outside, flaky-tender-inside pieces of fish. The only sounds were sighs of pleasure. Finally sated, they relaxed with cigarettes and the gourmet coffee from that battered old pot. Greg lit a cigar.

Greg hadn't been much of a smoker, but he usually enjoyed one after dinner. Floy had made him dispose of the remains someplace outside. The juniper bush by the front door didn't seem to mind.

Floy smoked. She'd started when she was 14, she'd told him, because all the flappers she saw in movies waved cigarettes in elegant long holders and at 14, every girl wants to look grown up. Half a pack a day—she rationed them.

She had assured him that her smoking had nothing to do with the colon cancer, and surgery had taken care of that problem. And he knew that she firmly believed her digestive system had been aided by her daily five o'clock libation.

He remembered that, after Florence Willoughby's comment about Floy's "great big drinks" (beer) compared to her "itty bitty" Manhattans, Floy had quit the beer, but the doctor okayed one drink a day, so at five o'clock every afternoon—she and Greg watched the clock carefully—she poured herself a generous double shot of Black Velvet, slightly diluted with 7-Up, while Greg fixed himself a bourbon, or, rarely, scotch. He didn't care for rye whiskey.

Greg had avoided any kind of liquor for a long time; he had vowed he would not be like his father. Then he began to realize that Mike and many of his other friends drank at times, but never turned into mean, sullen sourpusses. He came to enjoy a social drink or two with friends and with his wife. He didn't think he ever overdid it, not with Floy raising her eyebrows if he suggested "just freshening my drink a bit."

If he closed his eyes, Greg could imagine sitting outside the cottage with Floy, enjoying their pre-dinner drinks while trying out the new lawn chairs he'd just bought from one of the craft shops in town.

He had admired the master craftsmanship evident in those chairs, and in many of the pieces of furniture in the park, especially in the lightly wooded area crisscrossed with pebbled paths leading to the vast public beach and the main pier. There were benches and stools and window frames for the utilitarian park buildings and the museum, chairs and tables, big and small, in the buildings as well as glassed-in, wood-framed display cases.

He remembered seeking out the artist, for no crude carpentry had created such things—beautiful, useful, invisible to those who used them. He had met Mr. Green at his home, and had felt warmed by the pure kindness on that wrinkle-seamed old face with the young eyes. He remembered explaining that he had wanted to meet the creator of park benches that were so much more than park benches.

Later, he understood the frustration of a man whose income depended on producing and repairing purely useful things of wood that, in most park settings, were as rough and unattractive as old saw horses. Mr. Green's gift was transforming a once-living, once majestic tree, now a sad, stripped log, into a new shape, to live again in beauty.

Mr. Green's home was filled with tables, chairs, storage boxes, lamps, headboards, dressers, bureaus, and buffets, some with intricate carving, many polished to a high sheen but left to show the sheer complexity of the wood itself. Greg spent three hours examining the detail work and asking the questions that kept Mr. Green describing and demonstrating what he did. Greg could have stayed forever, but Floy would be wondering where he was.

As he was leaving, he finally dared to ask what had been lurking in his head since he had walked in the door—would Mr. Green teach him woodworking? He feared the inevitable answer would have to be a regretful "sorry, but I haven't the time." He remembered nothing of the drive home, just the euphoria of acceptance.

His first project, initially disappointing because he thought it would be too easy, too plain, too ordinary, was a little round stool, actually an old nail keg, looking like a little barrel with a plain circle for its top, with the sides wrapped in twine. It took hours to get that wood circle perfectly round and perfectly smooth before Mr. Green announced that it was ready for the varnish.

Greg was dismayed—and his face showed it—when Mr. Green told him that when the first coat of varnish was completely dry, Greg would sand it all off, back down to the bare wood, and then re-varnish. And then do it again. Only then would it be ready for the second and third coats of varnish, with light sanding and careful buffing between coats. But when it was done, a hand slowly skimmed over the surface revealed no bumps, no brush bristles trapped forever to mar the glass-smooth finish.

The next project was a drop-leaf table for breakfasts in the cottage kitchen. This time, Greg's face revealed only enthusiasm, not disappointment, at being told how to do what previously he might have thought an easy, slap-dash job. The twinkly young eyes in the crevassed old face laughed with him: "You're learning, young Greg. A drop-leaf table is not—or should not be—a rickety affair prone to collapsing just in time to dump the contents of a meal onto unwary diners' laps."

The simple, plain, understated elegance of that table, sitting quietly folded in a corner with a vase of wildflowers on a doily when not in use, almost made Greg preen. Unfolded, without a betraying creak or hitch or failure to support the necessities of an entire dinner for four or more people, it provided a serene backdrop for Floy's new cottage china—the moss-green and white stoneware with rustic patterns.

Under Mr. Green's tutelage, Greg made other things that summer: a small side-table with a very simple, very elegant oval top, an elaborately carved chair, end tables for books and magazines, and whimsical door handles for every door in the cottage.

One evening, toward the end of that magical summer, Mr. Green asked Greg, "Do you need a lamp? I've had this diamond willow sapling waiting for the right project, and I've been reluctant to cut it up. Just as it is, with a half-log as a base, it would be a beautiful floor lamp. It's yours, if you want it."

Want it? Greg coveted it! Whorls and knots, nearly black, embedded in the gold of the waiting tree, he could see the lamp it would be. And that was what Mr. Green had been teaching him: to visualize in memory, and to mourn, the death of a vibrant, breath-taking, beautiful tree, and not just imagine, but see, really see, what wasn't yet there, but would be, its forever-preserved essence. Was that, perhaps, what God saw in him?

15

HOME

Greg didn't remember that his 87th birthday had just passed. He had visitors. Some part of his brain recognized them as people who loved him, people he loved. That old lady: was she his mother? She was old. Then a synapse kicked in—he was old, too. His wife? Too hard to puzzle it out. That one looked like his wife as he remembered her, but she also looked like an older version of the daughter who used to go for horseback rides with him. No matter, she was smiling and hugging him, and he hugged back, also smiling. Whoever she was, he loved her.

The young one, the blond. Too old to be the little granddaughter who'd been at the lake one summer, but sure looked like her. She was smiling and hugging him, and this time, he found the words: "Cathy came?"

They—or the memories of them, which kept shifting from young bride and mother to older lifemate, from awkward coltish girl who knew how to sit a horse to the bride in her wedding finery he gave away to a man he did not like, from two-year-old charmer in her flannel nightie that her grandma had made to young woman with a two-year old of her own—they stayed with him all that day, and all that night. He felt the memory of his son's hands, so big and so gentle, and his baby daughter's tears, warm mist upon his face. The next morning, his chest hurt, and the white coats came, and all went dark. And then his mother was there to take him home, to the light.

AFTERWORD

Memories are founded on facts, but memories are not facts. They are the way an individual has shaped, altered, and refined factual chronologies, conversations, sights, feelings, and events. Memories are as true as facts, but in a different way. The creation of Mooswa is fact. There was a parade at the time. Greg's memory linked the two.

Greg's memories are true. Some of them are second-hand, comprised of conversations with the man himself, his family, friends, and hired companions, remembered and recorded by someone else. Some of the memories are first hand, from people like me who shared conversations and events with Greg.

For narrative purposes, to make <u>Try to Remember</u> Greg's story, not stories about him told by others, all the memories emanate from his mind, over the six years between the Alzheimer's diagnosis and his death.

The book was nearly finished when an article appeared, offering hope that Greg might actually have remembered thoughts and events long after it was assumed he could not. "[A]t any stage of dementia there is a range of capability. If you give people...activities that engage them...they come alive for the moment." ("Lost and Found" by Barbara Basler, quoting Dr. Cameron Camp, a research psychologist studying Alzheimer's, <u>AARP Bulletin</u>, September 2005.)

For Greg, talking to people was an activity that engaged him his entire life. Although the disease progressed inexorably and the moments when he came alive grew shorter and less frequent, asking him "Do you remember...?" often triggered another story.

Greg did converse during the first three years in the nursing home, often repeating himself, sometimes adding more details. For most of the fourth year, he responded to questions. The memories of the last year may not have been in his conscious mind at the time. I have assumed they could have been. I hope they were. His last clear statement is fact, and a cherished memory for me.

I am Greg's daughter. I am Judie.

978-0-595-37844-9
0-595-37844-7

www.ingramcontent.com/pod-product-compliance
Lightning Source LLC
Chambersburg PA
CBHW051422280526
45785CB00003B/1129